LOOKING GOOD
Is the Best Revenge

LOOKING GOOD

Is the Best Revenge

by

LINDA STASI

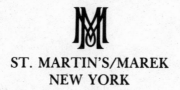

ST. MARTIN'S/MAREK
NEW YORK

Design by Laura Hammond

Library of Congress Cataloging in Publication Data

Stasi, Linda.
    Looking good is the best revenge.

    1. Beauty, Personal.   2. Women—Health and hygiene.
I. Title.
RA778.S7957   1984   646.7'0088042   83–21214
ISBN 0–312–49812–8

First Edition
10 9 8 7 6 5 4 3 2 1

For R.P.M.
without whom this book
would not have been written . . .
in fact,
it wouldn't even have been necessary!

"Honey, no matter what he says,
it's *always* a toots!"
Florence Stasi . . . 1977, 1978, 1979, etc.

Contents

Acknowledgments

Thank you: Julia Coopersmith, my agent, who said, "My God! That's a book title!" Joyce Engelson, my editor, who said, "You're right, that *is* a book title!" Deborah Daly, who believed in this project from day one and who worked so hard to make it look like it sounds. Roni Feldblum, who typed and sorted a massive amount of cross-out pages. Annette Capone, Sally Horton, Edy Krauss, Barbara Gordon, Stuart Berger, Nancy Hissom, Sandy Boylan, Gail Yancosek, Janet Kurzweil, Don & Gloria Stasi, and Joe Saffon for giving freely of their love, support, and knowledge whenever I needed it.

And finally, to my daughter Jessica, who let me use her room and mess it up with typewriters, papers, and notes without complaining. Much.

LOOKING GOOD
Is the Best Revenge

1 · Why Is Looking Good the Best Revenge?

There is only one thing more certain than death and taxes: You never feel dumpier than when you've been dumped. Any woman who has ever been dumped by any man, rejected by any person, place, or thing, knows how true this is. True, but not necessary. There is also another truth: Looking good is the *best* revenge.

When is looking good the best revenge? When you meet the bum after a few months and you look gorgeous and his girlfriend is such a dog that her name should be Spot! Or when you go to your high school reunion and the ex-prom queen *is* the class float because she weighs 9000 pounds. Or when your ex-husband comes to pick the kids up for the weekend and you are dressed to kill (him?) for your date with the world's handsomest man.

And that's what this book is all about: feeling awful and looking wonderful! They really aren't mutually exclusive, you know. In fact, it *is* possible to feel like two cents and look like a million. It's all a matter of what you do to and with yourself after you have decided to take to your bed.

So, you see, this is a beauty book, and a feel better book, but its main purpose is to give you what you really want—revenge. In it you will find lots of ways to get gorgeous, get thin, and get even!! But right off the bat, let me tell you that I won't force you to go out, socialize, get a new job, or anything. In fact, I think that you should be allowed to stay home as much as you want, feel sorry for yourself, sleep a lot, use up massive amounts of Kleenex®, cry over old mementos and become an absolute bore to at least one good friend.

Why? Because a good reactive depression (one that is caused by a truly lousy event, rather than one that is chronic) takes anywhere from about two months to one year to go and find itself another home. While it is inhabiting *your* body, however, I think that you should be allowed to indulge yourself shamelessly. After all, you've worked for it, and you deserve it. But, you should be forced into knowing that when this crummy period passes, and it will, you can end up:

1. Thinner

2. Prettier

3. Smarter

4. Sexier

Remember, sooner or later you will run into Mr. Once-Was-Wonderful. How you put yourself back together will drive him wild and make you feel terrific. While he's been partying, you've been rejuvenating. He will look dissipated and you, divine. You will be five pounds thinner, your skin will be glowing, and your hair will be shining.

And *that's* what this book is all about . . . using this time to get gorgeous. Yes, you'll find tons of make-at-home and do-at-home facials, hair conditioners, and diet tips and tricks, but they'll be based on indulging yourself. And remember, too, that there are several benefits, beyond simple revenge, for using this time to indulge yourself. One is that you won't feel guilty about wanting to lie around the house, and the second is that people will begin to tell you how you've never looked better in your life. It's amazing how that alone can give you a major boost, when you know in your heart you feel like a frog.

Yes, Virginia, there is an end to everything . . . including obsessional love affairs and feeling rotten. With any luck it will happen sooner than later for you. But in the meantime, read on. You'll not only learn how to look better, but you'll have something to read while you're lying around the house waiting for the phone to ring.

2 · No! You're Not Crazy, You're Just Feeling Bad!

Whatever it is that has caused you to feel so awful, remember that unless you are Mrs. Haversham and have chosen to sit around in your wedding gown for the rest of your life, you will feel better again. It won't happen today, however. And in our society where instant gratification (to be henceforth known as instant grats) is what we expect (though seldom ever get), it becomes pretty difficult to understand that unless it happens immediately, it will ever happen at all.

Feeling better takes time. Sometimes two weeks, sometimes a year. But it will happen. And it's okay to feel angry, sad, crummy and generally sexless. (No, abstinence does *not* make the heart—or the libido—grow fonder. In fact, it often makes you totally abstinenced minded!) But the one thing that it's *not* okay to feel is helpless. You aren't. Although we are brought up to believe that life "ain't worth a damn without a man," it ain't necessarily so. But, like it or not, there *will* be other men. In fact, some of them may even make you feel bad *again,* and you may make some of *them* feel bad again. It's just the way it is.

And, I can also say from experience, that there may be several one-and-onlys in your life. It's just that each time that special magic happens between you and someone else, you forget that it has happened before and that it can—and will—happen to you again. While that may not be earth-shattering news, it *is* necessary that somewhere in your psyche you believe it.

And it is necessary, too, that sometime in the not-too-distant future, you set about making it happen. I don't recommend that you go out and try to make it happen today, however. Today is wrong, but in a few weeks or months, it *will* be right.

Why is it wrong, now? Because now you are probably feeling very low on self-esteem. And when you are feeling low, you can very easily blow it with men whom you may not enjoy now, but may enjoy several months from now. And another thing, if you are still enamored of Mr. Once-Was, you'll be so busy comparing the two men that you'll never enjoy Mr. Almost-but-Not-Quite-As-Wonderful.

Let me tell you what happened to me. I'm laughing about it now. (Well, almost laughing; let's call it a large smirk.) After my major obsessional love affair—which was even more traumatic for me than getting divorced—I decided that I should go out with lots of men. In the first five months, I dated about ten men. I hated them all. Or was repulsed by them all. Why? Were they dumpy, creepy androids who wanted me to split the bill for burgers? Did they wear short black socks with large Bermuda shorts, or get up and sing "My Way" at family weddings? Hardly. They were some of the most fantastic bachelors in New York City. There were several very handsome doctors, two best-selling authors, a few independently wealthy men (who seemed just to read the *Wall Street Journal* and be driven around by their drivers all day), a carpenter with a Ph.D. (who sailed his boat from New England to New York, docked it next to my apartment building and refused to leave unless I saw him), and one desperado filmmaker.

Given the opportunity to redo what I blew, I'd keep every one of these men on hold, for at *least* a few months. I wasn't ready. I'd go out on dates, forcing myself to go because that's what the books and the shrinks say should be done. But each time I'd go, I'd feel like crying. There I'd be, sitting in a lovely restaurant with a gorgeous man, and all I wanted to do was to go home, forget about the wining and dining and get on with the plain old whining! Crazy? No. I just wasn't ready.

I would end up telling each of my dates all about my broken love affair. And guess what? I'm sure they ended up feeling as though I *did* think of them as creepy androids with short black socks. And, even though I was the one who broke up my previous affair, I was in the pits about it for months. It wasn't until I gave it up emotionally that I was ready to go out and enjoy myself with other men. Of course, by that time, I'd already met and ruined my chances with every available friend of a friend in town. I'd wiped out my resources!!

So, be careful, and don't force yourself to go out too soon. And, if all else fails, be honest! Tell any man who asks you out that you just aren't seeing *anyone* these days. But also say that when you *are* ready to to out again, *you'd* love to give *him* a call. This answer not only keeps you from an uncomfortable situation, it seems to drive men wild. I have found that men react to this answer by sticking to you like white on rice. Each one thinks that he is the one who can change your celibate state. You not only get to do what *you* want to do, but you become very mysterious, desirable, and sought-after in the bargain. It's really quite wonderful. But even if they *don't* call you, do call each of them. When you are ready. And not a moment before that.

You'll see. They will be very flattered and you will have a pocketful of numbers before long. If, however, you really don't think that a particular man is for you—now or ever—take his number anyway. Give it to a friend. Let her have him, because he might be just perfect for her, if not for you. One word of caution here: Don't go out with him first, under any circumstances, because then you just *can't* give him away. He will feel rejected and dumb, and your friend will think she's getting your leftovers. If, on the other hand, you think that perhaps you just don't like him *now* because you are depressed, keep that number all to yourself. And do call.

Now, what about that depression? Do you feel as though no one in the world has ever felt as badly as you are feeling right now? Have you suddenly decided that the only real truth and beauty in the world lies in the lyrics of country/western music? Does it feel as though walking and breathing at the same time is a major accomplishment? Well, take solace in the fact that you are not alone. Millions of people are feeling just what you are feeling right now. And here's the good news: Millions more have felt exactly this same way in the past and don't anymore.

In fact, estimates by the National Institute of Mental Health indicate that fifteen percent of adults between eighteen and seventy-four may suffer from severe depressions in any given year. Now, some of those people, are of course, chronically depressed, and need professional help right away. But many of them are having reactive depressions.

So, how do you know that *your* depression is not the kind that will last forever? You don't really know that for sure, but you *can* get a pretty good indication that it won't last by the mere fact that you are reading this book. You obviously *do* want to look and feel better. And looking good and feeling great are important decisions that a person must make, if she is to take charge. In fact, one of the first signs that a psychiatrist will look for in a depressed patient is how the patient cares for herself physically. A person who is severely depressed just doesn't care, generally, how she looks. Her hair is unkempt, her clothes are thrown on haphazardly, her whole demeanor is one of disarray and lack of concern. You, on the other hand, *want* to look and feel better. And this book is going to help you to do just that.

If, however, your depression doesn't seem to be lifting *at all* (after a few weeks, or a few months at the most), it's time to get professional help. Most larger cities have Depression Studies programs and centers, which are usually located in university medical centers. The doctors who staff these programs are trained to deal specifically with depression and they are the tops in their field. Don't be afraid to call for help if you need it.

But remember, you should allow yourself to feel sad, unhappy, and upset for a *time*—without getting panicky. Even Freud wrote, in *Mourning and Melancholia,* that a person must go through a sad period before seeing the light again. And that's just what this period is for you, a period of mourning . . . whether you are mourning the loss of a lover, the loss of a job, or the loss of your pride. It may be surprising to you, in fact that you are feeling sad (which seems inappropriate) when you should be feeling angry (which seems appropriate). Well, depression *has* been called rage turned inward. And that seems right to me. I mean, let's face it, you can't go out and yell at the world without being put away (or worse, without becoming humiliated), so you turn it inward. And guess who inward is? I'll give you a hint: It's the one person who is guaranteed to share your bed and bath—forever.

But now we're about to change that. Because if you remember nothing else, you must remember this one thing: Revenge is sweeter than *any* embarrassing rage you can ever hurl at Mr. Once-Was-Wonderful. And the best revenge? Your own happiness, of course. And it's a happiness that comes from within you . . . and a happiness that will show *all* over (the outside of) you!

Oh yes, a footnote here. Remember me telling you about my Mr. Once-Was-Wonderful? The one I anguished over for months? (Seven, to be exact.) Well, when I finally decided that he was old news, I found a new Mr. Wonderful-Dashing-Desperado. We were riding in a convertible on an island in New England one sunny Saturday, with a carload of little kids, my daughter included. When what to my wondering eyes should appear? A great big green jeep and one lousy old flame! And *he* was alone! It couldn't have been a better scenario if I'd written it myself: There I was with the world's handsomest man (well, almost) and a car full of gorgeous kids. And I must say, I was tan and trim and feeling terrific at the time myself!

Ah, revenge is sweet! And guess what? I never once, not once, regretted having spent seven months of my life lying around my apartment feeling sorry for myself. I learned, after all, to cry without wrecking my eyes, and how to make the most of the time I spent hiding out. And so will you.

Now . . . let's start plotting your *beautiful* revenge!

3 · Bed and Bored? The Truth about Taking to Your Bed

Okay, it's true. It's happened. You don't want to get out of bed. When you are at work, all you think about is the weekend. No, not for the fun you'll have, but for the opportunity it will afford you to take to your bed. (Freedom to lie there with the covers pulled up over your ears, no doubt.)

Is this, you wonder, what the rest of your life is going to be like, all tears and no cheers? Are you doomed to a life lived under the covers? Are you going quite mad, like a stricken heroine in a gothic novel? No, to the first, no to the second, and definitely no to the last. You are just feeling rotten, miserable, and out of touch with everything but the ache. That's okay, really it is. It's actually healthier than not dealing with it and pretending that everything is wonderful. If you don't allow yourself to get over the pain, you won't be able to go on to the happiness.

When can you expect the ache to dull, and the laughs to begin? Well, it depends on you . . . and on your particular situation. But sooner or later, within a few weeks, or a few months, you will bottom out. Then suddenly you will find that you want to go out. You will also find that several hours have passed without a thought of Mr. Once-Was-Wonderful, or even a thought about the pain. You will *even* find, much to your surprise, that you've managed a whole conversation without mentioning your dilemma, even once. But it will take time.

Why the bed, though? Think about this: Isn't your bed the closest you will ever come to the safety and shelter of the womb? Now, that's *really* going home to mother . . . the mother who was all accepting, all protecting, nonjudgmental. The very thing we all wanted, and the very thing that *no* human being can ever be. Remember, while you may have an extremely supportive mother, she still has a vested interest—you. And that makes her judgmental. As much as she may try to keep quiet, she just won't be able to resist saying that she never did see what you saw in him or that he *always was* a "womanizer," low life, a snob, a bum, or an arrogant S-O-B. And then you'll feel worse. Much worse.

The other reason I think we like to take to our beds is that it's a place to go through withdrawal without more pain in the brain. I mean, they give drug addicts padded cells, don't they? The least you can give yourself is a padded bed to thrash about in. And, let's admit it. A major obsessional affair is like an addiction. You only feel lit up and high when you are talking to, seeing, feeling your lover. Everything else seems immaterial to that high. If it's an out-of-control obsession, you may even feel that everything that happens to you in life only happens so that you can share it with him.

Let's take Mara, for example. Mara is a freelance writer. One day she was assigned to interview a famous author for a magazine article. When she walked into his office, the magic happened. Unfortunately, the magician was married. But that didn't stop them. And although Mara managed to keep the interview very businesslike, there was enough electricity flying around the room to light up Detroit. When the interview ended, Mara, with shaking knees, got up to shake his hand. As she reached out to take his hand, he swept her up and gave her the most passionate kiss she'd ever had. She kissed back. And that, as they say, was that. She was hooked on an addiction. Incredible as it sounds, within weeks the magician even left his hearth and home. He said he couldn't bear to be without Mara, and couldn't bear the thought of her with another man. He was constantly in touch with her . . . emotionally and physically . . . for two years. She helped him with the most minute details of his divorce, she tended to his tender feelings, she helped him make the transition from husband to (she hoped) husband. His divorce took two years to complete. And guess what he did to celebrate? He moved in with another woman!

It took Mara a good six months to come to grips with the fact that she was not his end, she was just his means. He had wanted to get a divorce, but lacked the courage and Mara was simply his excuse. He is the type of man who can't be without a relationship for two seconds!

Mara got all of the pent-up passion (good and bad), all of the nitty-gritty day-to-day details, all of the major problems of his life. And when he was finally over the divorce part of his life, he was ready to start anew. But not alone. He chose a woman, totally unlike Mara in every way. While Mara was passionate, loving, and concerned, this new woman was socially correct, cold, and aloof. Just like the ex-wife who had supposedly made him "so unhappy."

Mara, of course, took to her bed (as any self-respecting woman would). The withdrawal was hard. She wept over his old letters and photos. She wrote reams of purple prose. She bored her friends to tears over every contact she subsequently had with her ex-lover. She looked for clues that he really didn't mean it . . . and for clues that would indicate his sudden return.

After six months, she began to see two things very clearly: One was that she was never the woman he would end up with because, quite frankly, the man just would never belong to any club that would have him for a member. Mara not only had made him a member of her club, she'd made him president! His post-deb, on the other hand, was too busy getting her nails done to notice that he could, would, or should even dare to have problems.

The other insight that she had (after a long haul) was one that *could* have come from her mother. She just didn't know what she saw in him in the first place! He wasn't nice, or especially interesting . . . he was just great in bed. It took her awhile to realize that great sex does not always equal great love.

Mara recovered in the same way that you will. She took to her bed, did a lot of thinking, and a lot of recuperating. She also spent that time experimenting with her hair, her face, and her body. When she was feeling especially miserable, she'd give herself a facial, when she was feeling drained, she energized with exercises, when she was feeling ugly, she did something terrific to her hair. She revamped her wardrobe, experimented with new ways to wear old clothes (after all, she didn't want to go shopping, God knows), and began slowly to look completely different. Her depression-induced lethargy actually gave her a chance to unwind, explore, and finally emerge—a beauty! While she was always attractive, now she was a knockout. While she had always dressed and fixed herself in a neat, conservative way, she now went a little wild. After all she'd had months of experimenting! All of that time she'd spent hiding out wasn't, as her friends feared, ruining her . . . it was revamping her. And guess what? She met more men, had more dates, and even got her chance, when the time came, to reject her old lover! When they met a year later he went wild over the "new" confident Mara. She, however, was on to a better more stable relationship by then.

So accept the fact that the time you will spend hiding out isn't *wasted time.* It's necessary time. Time you allow yourself to think out, play out, and feel out all of those tangled emotions. And while it's true that Mara's profession allowed her more time to take to her bed than most people will ever have, you can do it too. *You* know when it's feasible and when it's not. I don't have to tell you that. You deserve it, you need it, and you want it. Just don't feel guilty about it. It's a great way to discover that you *too* deserve better than what you've allowed yourself to have.

Now, let's get on with it. This, dear heart, is going to be something completely different! I won't force you to do one thing that you don't want to do. *You* will choose to do this or that, and soon enough, you'll be wanting to do more and more and then you'll start wanting to get out more and more. But for now? Do exactly as you please. After all, no one should be forced to go to a Georgette Klinger Salon with tears streaming down her face!

Okay, now that you've taken to your bed, I'm not

going to tell you not to think about *him* . . . not yet anyway. In fact, now's the time to take a look at that man. Yes, it's true, you're going to find him right here on the next few pages. And I'm sure you'll be shocked to discover that he's not unique at all. . . .

4 · Over and Out

Okay, you're saying to yourself, this is all well and good, but will it ever *really* be over and done with? Will I ever stop thinking about him? Well, the truth is that even if you *are* saying to yourself, "But I still feel rotten!," you will also see that whole hours will pass by soon without even a thought of Mr. Once-Was. And one of these days you will also see that you felt worse yesterday. Time is what will really heal you . . . this time that you are using right now. So let's make it count. No, I'm not going to lecture you or make you do anything that you don't want to do, but I am going to try to help you figure out where you went wrong last time out.

Now, let's think about just *why* your last affair went bad, and what you can do the next time out to prevent a rehash of the same old thing. You see, chances are good, that unless you honestly know what went wrong, you will let all of this new gorgeousness you are going to experiment with—as soon as you can get up enough energy to sit up—go to waste. Why will it go to waste? Because you might just do the same thing all over again. We do tend to stick to what we know . . . no matter how crummy it feels. So, let's get a grip on the situation and you can mull it around while you're lying around.

Is it the men you choose? Probably. If you look closely you may even see a pattern emerging. Are you after the elusive desperado? Or maybe it's Mama's favorite son, or the forever married man, or even the profoundly uncommitted man. Not one of these men is ever going to make you happy. But they do, after all, have their own special brand of appeal. Let's take a closer look at each type. And remember, if this man didn't make you happy, (although he claimed to love you), the problem is really with him. And take great solace in the fact that he's not going to run off and be happy with someone else (even though he may indeed run off and make someone else crazy). It's not *just* you. And guess what? If he can't commit himself to someone he *loves,* which he probably can't, than *he's* the one who will be ultimately unhappy.

5 · Wanted Dead or Alive: The Four Most Elusive Types of Men

When wizened old women sit around the campfire telling stories of the big ones that got away, they inevitably tell tales of the big four.

The big four are the elusive ones . . . the ones who seem so right for you. And yet somehow it just never works out. You are probably recovering from one of these guys right now. You might even have been married to one.

You've gone through the whole thing in your mind a hundred times. You feel that it's your fault . . . maybe if you'd just been prettier, smarter, more experienced, less experienced . . . better. Maybe then he would have stayed.

Guess what? It's not your fault. No one is pretty enough, smart enough, or has the right amount of experience for these guys. So, while you can't change what's happened in the past, you can control what happens to you in the future.

Here, then is a rundown of the big four . . . the ones who always seem to get away. But now you'll be the one who gets away . . . and the one who's in control. Remember, even if he left you for another woman, he won't change. But you *will.* Now you'll know what to look out for . . . and you'll have the goods on the next one who shows up. And trust me, another one will show up. Just keep in mind that it's better to know them than to loathe them.

Here are the warning signs:

THE DESPERADO

Physical Description

Handsome in an offbeat way, swaggers without meaning to, can be tall, short, dark, light, and everything in between. His distinguishing characteristics are eyes that laugh the minute he meets you, clothes that would probably look dumb on anyone else, and an assurance so complete you immediately want to make love to him or drown him.

His Opening Remarks

"You really are quite a beautiful woman. I noticed you the second you walked into the room . . . let's get out of here." He may (or may not) give you the most unwholesome kiss you've ever had.

Your Opening Remarks

"I'd love to, but I'm going to a Junior League benefit with Prince Rainier."

Physical Afflictions

The need to wear baseball caps, jeans, and handmade jackets. He also knows the best tailors, the best barbers (this one wouldn't be caught dead having his hair cut by a "stylist"), and is on a personal basis with ticket scalpers, gamblers, the social elite, and artists. He has the uncanny ability to recite unexpurgated Chaucer while beating up street toughs, and is comfortable playing football, tennis, squash, and poker with the pros. He can also cook up a gourmet meal that will knock your socks off.

His M.O.

The man is unique. (Or so it seems.) He will sweep you off your feet, make hours of love to you, make you feel as though he's never met anyone on earth who even compares to you. He will ask you to go away with him on your first date . . . not because he's dying to take you away . . . but just to find out where he stands with you. He calls three, four, five times a day, sends you flowers at work with outrageous cards that make you blush, takes you to the opera, the ballet, and the prize fights. When you go out with his friends you never know whether you will be with a movie producer, an ex-girlfriend, the Pope, or a gangster. He is irresistible. And he makes you feel the same way. He is monogamous. For short periods of time.

Then he decides that you just aren't nice, kind, funny, or adventurous enough. And guess what? In two seconds he has found yet another one and only. He is monogamous: As in serial monogamy.

Your M.O.

If you really can't resist desperados, then you must never let them know it. You must appear to be better than they are, unappreciative of any and all gestures, and you must also constantly send yourself flowers. Tell him that you sent them to yourself, and he will go crazy with jealousy. He will be sure that you've made up an awful lie. This can, of course, become quite tedious and expensive. If you can give yourself a title of some minor importance, such as the granddaughter of the deposed Lord of Stratfordhaven, you've got him for life. If you can't meet all of the above qualifications, however, it's best to steer clear. This one is armed and very dangerous. But, boy, is he great in bed!

HARRY, THE ETERNALLY MARRIED MAN

Physical Description

A sad look around the eyes that comes from living with a wife who doesn't understand him (not to mention too many years of arguing with Little League coaches). His clothing is conservative (as befits a husband), and his briefcase is large. It often contains a duplicate shirt of the one he left the house with this morning. (It wouldn't do to go home with lipstick and perfume on his collar, now, would it?)

His Opening Remarks

"It's tough to live in a marriage with a woman you no longer love and no longer sleep with."

Your Opening Remarks

"Did you know the latest statistics show that only fifty percent of all married people sleep together? It seems that all of the wives sleep with their husbands and none of the husbands sleep with their wives."

Physical Afflictions

The map of Larchmont, Greenwich, or Shaker Heights tattooed on his forehead, a monthly commuter ticket stuck to his heart, and the fear of turning into a pumpkin if he misses the 10:05 train home.

His M.O.

Within the first half hour of meeting you he will tell you that (1) He is married and (2) He never cheats on his wife. The third thing he will do is try to madly seduce you while proclaiming that he's never done this sort of thing before (well, at least not before the last time and the time before that).

Your M.O.

If you must go out with him, realize that he probably won't leave his hearth and home for you. And even if he does, he will only discover what freedom is like after you've nursed him through his divorce. Keep dating every other man in the world, drive him wild with jealousy, and break many dates with him (even if it kills you). Never let him know that you aren't seeing anyone else. And, in reality, try not ever to let that happen. Your only protection against Harry is to date other men. If you can date him without becoming obsessed, it's okay. But if you think that the affair will turn into a major obsession, run, walk, split, take off for the hills, and get out of there.

You really don't need to spend Christmas, Thanksgiving, Arbor Day, and the Washington's birthday weekend alone, you know.

THE PROFOUNDLY UNCOMMITTED MAN

Physical Description

Always in a starched shirt and impeccably pressed clothing. He can be tall, short, exciting, or boring. The most distinguishing physical characteristic, however, is his unrivaled ability to make confirmed plans with his friends for all vacations, summers, and holidays years in advance, while being unable to make future plans with you that extend beyond the next fifteen minutes.

His Opening Remarks

"I've just never found a woman who could be all of the things that I need. I guess I'm just too tough, but God, I'd love to be married, have kids, you know, the whole nine yards."

Your Opening Remarks

"If there's anything on earth that I don't want to be it's married! Why do I only meet men who want to get married? It's very tough, you know."

Physical Afflictions

An addiction to good stereo equipment, natural fibers, and his cleaning lady. He has never seen the inside of a laundry room, an oven, or a station wagon. He may never be stylish, but he is *clean.* In point of fact, no woman can ever compare to his cleaning lady for sheer competence.

His M.O.

He will call you up, ask you for a date, and you will have a very special and lovely time together. He may not call you again. But if he does, it won't be right away, it won't be regular, and it won't be often. It's not that he has millions of other women, it's just that he has plans. Always. Even if his plans are merely to install yet another tweeter, they are *his* plans and he wouldn't think of changing them. He also can't think of marrying you . . . or anyone else . . . because he's already planned to take a house in the Hamptons this summer with a group of friends, and then there's his Club Med trip in the fall and then. . . .

Your M.O.

Tell him you're busy the first time he calls, and the second. On the third call, accept his date and then spend a lot of time leaving the table to go to the phone. Call the weather if you have no one else to call, but don't give him your full attention. Get an answering machine, and leave it on at night. You may not win him, but at least he'll know that there does exist a woman with . . . plans.

MAMA'S FAVORITE SON

Physical Description

Handsome in a wimpish kind of way, charming, and very sweet. Or so it seems. Even if he has managed to get his own place, he visits his mother often. And well. His clothing is often an embarrassingly bad attempt at "hipness," but his sensitivity shines through. After all, who can think badly of a man who will give up a Saturday to clean his mother's clogged leaders and gutters?

His Opening Remarks

"It's really nice to meet an old-fashioned girl." (You will never be a woman to this one!) "It's so rare today to meet someone with your kinds of qualities. Do you live with your parents?"

Your Opening Remarks

"Yes, I am old fashioned . . . I still prefer sex with men to sex with women, electronic devices, and sheep. I got my own place fifteen years ago. Whom do you live with?"

His M.O.

He will take you to dinner at his mother's house. She will fuss over you and make you feel special. She will, in fact, make you feel so right for her son. Then she will knife you in the back. She will tell him that she's heard that women of your religion sleep with sheep. He will grudgingly see that Mama was right all along. You will never get him to marry you until she dies. But then it's better than getting him to marry you just when she gets around to needing a full-time nurse.

Your M.O.

Be exactly the opposite of his mother. Be a sex fiend who can never get enough of him. Send him erotic chocolates and take him away to a nude beach. Tell him you like his mother, but don't go with him when he visits. Let them beg. Drive him wild, and do disappear from time to time. Even Mama will pale under this onslaught.

Then marry someone else. He will never change and you will never learn to make beef stew like you know who!

6 · Stop Being So Grateful! (How to Succeed with Men without Really Trying)

Aside from looking out for the wrong types of men, how do you guarantee—or at least place the odds in your favor—that you won't blow it when a nice man does come along? Well, first of all, you can begin to unlearn a lot of the patterns that it took you years to build up. And lying around in your bed is the best place to do just that.

Now, don't get nervous. I'm not going to lecture you, or tell you what you should have done in the past to prevent how you are feeling now. I *am* going to tell you that it's fine that you are going to use this time to learn how *not* to be the next time.

So what's the secret besides avoiding the BIG FOUR? For one thing, stop being so damn grateful for every little thing that he does. Remember, you deserve to be treated well and even if he *is* a nice guy, you won't catch him acting grateful because he's found you. Ever.

Well, I honestly believe that before the last decade (when women started panicking because they suddenly discovered that there were more of us then there are of them), we were much better off. Women used to be chased by men, women used to leave men, women used to flirt outrageously with dozens of men and break hundreds of hearts. Now it's all turned around. Was it the sexual revolution (you know, the one that took the thrill out of the chase)? Maybe it was just that we were so busy trying to prove our equal status that we knocked 'em dead at work and began groveling at home! Well, get off your knees and take stock of yourself! Remember, you don't often find the wives who are getting their nails done (while their husbands are making excuses to you) groveling around!

There's no reason on earth to be grateful because he stays the night, eats your food, messes up your bathroom, and leaves at two the next afternoon. HE SHOULD BE GRATEFUL that you allowed him to stay as long as you did. It's your life, after all! Start acting as though you own it, and stop being grateful that he's chosen to use up a bit of it. Expect more and you'll get more. Don't be thrilled that he's asked you out. Are you such a dog, and he such a prince? Stop thinking that he's better than you, and that you're lucky just to have him. If you remember nothing else that you read in this book, remember that if *you* don't believe that *he's* a lucky man for finding *you*, he won't *either*.

The second thing we must stop doing is jumping into bed so easily. Yes. That *was* a revolutionary statement . . . but then I've never been known for my moderate views. What is it with us anyway? How can we possibly do the most intimate physical things with a man whom we are afraid to call the next day? It just doesn't make sense!

Think about it. Why should you spend the night with a man, not knowing if he will even call you again—and knowing that you aren't comfortable calling him? Yes, yes, I know all about how the experience is enough for a liberated woman. They tell us (the manifestos on such things) that sex is something that women are now free to indulge in whenever the urge strikes. Well, the truth is that the manifesto writers forgot about intimacy and friendship—which is ultimately what women want from men.

I really think that you've got to get to know him—and know him well—before you decide that you are going to get physical. While it seems all well and good that we are free to do whatever we want with whomever we want, the truth is that we just aren't that free. Most people—men and women—don't enjoy wham, bam, and so forth. If we *were* that free we wouldn't have the slightest hesitation about calling at any time, would we?

So, why not let *him* work at it again. Let him worry that you *won't* call him, rather than have him worry that you *will!* I, for one, will never allow myself to get crazed over someone I don't feel free to call. They don't worry about it ever, now do they? Why not let a relationship progress naturally, letting the sexual tension build? What's the big payoff anyway?

The third most important thing? Stop trying to be superwoman. Whoever said that you had to be the best at your job, at your sport, at mothering, and at every other thing you've ever attempted? In the last few years, we've begun to think that way. And feminists aside, a lot of it stems from wanting to shine with men. It really does.

It's back to that old feeling that if you want a man you've got to beat out the competition. You must be better at everything than anyone else. Not true.

Here's another story: Ann was dating a man who was quite attractive (not gorgeous), quite successful (because his family owned the world), and quite funny (*that* he came by naturally). They spent a lot of time together, and she thought that this was just terrific. But to win such a prize, she also thought that she had to be worthy of him. So she dazzled him with her amazing ability to run an advertising company, lecture on the college circuit, spend massive amounts of time with her son, and still be five minutes early for the ballet, looking great.

Instead of thinking that he should have been lucky to have found her, she thought that she was lucky to have found him. Why? What was so spectacular about him? If truth be told, her sense of humor was every bit as good as his, she came by her success honestly (not because it was bought for her), she raised a wonderful, funny child, and still managed to be a sexy, divorced mother.

Well, needless to say, Ann *was* grateful, so *he* wasn't. When they split up, because he had started to see someone else (she wasn't *that* grateful!), he told Ann that she (Ann) was a woman of rare quality and beauty and he loved her for it. Could it be? Had he been so fortunate to have found *two* women of rare quality and beauty? Hardly. What he *had* found was a woman who had put herself together well . . . but she was no natural beauty. She wasn't particularly funny, bright, or successful, either. So, what did she have that Ann didn't have? A lack of gratitude, that's what!

Ann did get her revenge though. A few months later they ran into each other at a party . . . or should I say, he saw Ann and ran away. The reason? Ann had bounced back, looking beautiful, and his girlfriend needed a leash to go out. He even called Ann a few days later. She told him that she was busy and would call him right back. He never heard from her again.

Now, collapse if you like . . . you've worked for it, and you deserve it.

7 · The Shameless Day Off: Indulge Yourself—It's Later Than You Think

Puritan ethics have taught us that there is something inherently wrong about wanting to spend a lot of time in bed alone. This common, every-night experience is turned into a terrible and degenerate experience when performed in the cold light of day. I think that is nonsense. I consider my bed a friend and I take to it whenever I feel bad. I have learned to do so without feeling guilty, although it took great amounts of time in bed feeling guilty to get over it.

We think, "Oh my God, I'm lying around like a slug when I could be out doing something productive." You *are* doing something productive: You are recuperating. You are indulging yourself. After all, no one else is going to indulge you now. The dashing desperado has left you high and dry, or has forced you to break it up, so you aren't about to get massive bunches of flowers.

But if you are so inclined, and if it will make you feel better, there are many useful and interesting things that you can do while lying around that will help you to look and feel better.

First, however, you must begin by taking a day off. And I don't mean a Saturday, when your kids may be home. I mean a day during the week, when you skip work. Yes, skip work just to indulge yourself. It doesn't feel nearly as good if you indulge yourself when you are supposed to. You wouldn't hesitate to take a day off if someone died or you were sick, would you? Then think of it as a day of mourning for your relationship and that you are sick about it. There, that should take care of the guilt!

Now that you've done it, enjoy it. Begin this day by staying in bed as long as you like. You need only get out to make yourself a light breakfast, which you will savor in bed, and to take yourself a long warm, fragrant bath, which you will savor for the pure luxury of it.

Let's start with breakfast. My favorite breakfast in bed consists of:

- A small pot of Celestial Seasonings non-caffeinated tea
- A container of yogurt sprinkled with wheat germ on top (it makes it seem like a fattening piece of pie)
- One mimosa (half a glass of orange juice mixed with half a glass of champagne)

But you can prepare whatever breakfast makes you feel most taken care of. This is not the day you will start your diet necessarily, or the day you will stick to it, if you really don't want to. This is your day just to indulge yourself.

After breakfast, take a second snooze. When you wake up, run a bath for yourself. Now you probably think that you know how to take a bath. Well, maybe you do and maybe you don't. I don't think that a bath is a place to lie around and get clean. You can get clean in the shower. A bath should be a luxurious beauty ritual that will leave you relaxed and smoother. Here are some of my favorite ways to do just that.

BATHING BEAUTIES

TEST THE TEMP

Did you know that bathwater that is too hot can dry out your skin, and can even be overstimulating? The ideal water for a good relaxing soak is between eighty-five and ninety-five degrees. So keep it at that temperature, if it's just relaxation you're after.

AT HOME SPA

Create your own spa shop at home by placing two towels on the radiator, out in the sun, or in a running dryer. If you use the dryer, or the sun, take them out just before you step into the bath, and keep them warm on the radiator (in winter) or on the open windowsill in the sun (in summer).

As your towels are heating up, run a bath using one of the formulas below. Rub your body down with a loofah or natural bristle brush to slough off dead skin, before you bathe. Wipe your body lightly with a fresh towel. Step in, place a rolled up towel under your head for comfort, and relax for about twenty minutes. Step out and lightly blot up dripping water with the first warmed towel. Slather up your still damp body with your favorite moisturizer, and wrap up in towel number two. You'll feel wonderful.

THE WATER WORKS . . . A BUNCH OF BEAUTY BATHS

WE CALL IT MAIZE BATH
To Smooth You

1 qt. whole milk
½ cup corn oil

Blend the corn oil and milk together and pour into a warm bath. Step in, relax, and enjoy all of that softness.

Take a Bath with Skin Care Expert Lia Schorr

Lia knows all about good times, hard times, and tense times. Here's how the lady who works twenty-eight hours a day relaxes in the bath.

GET LOOSE WITH JUICE BATH
To Rejuvenate Any Skin Type

You're feeling tense and uptight. Then loosen up and rev up by taking a dip in the "C!" This bath will not only cleanse you, and cool you off, but it will rejuvenate your skin . . . and maybe even your mood.

All you need to do is squeeze the juice from two fat oranges into a tub of lukewarm water. Then lie back and soak for about fifteen minutes. Step out and pat dry. The vitamin C will be absorbed by your skin making it—and you—feel invigorated.

BY THE SEA SALT BATH
To Nourish and Stimulate Your Tired Bod . . . and Skin

2 teaspoons sea salt
½ teaspoon lemon juice
1½ tablespoons sesame seed oil

Feeling unloved, unwanted, and generally lousy? Then indulge yourself by taking a seaside vacation . . . right in your own home. Here's how: Combine the ingredients, add them to your lukewarm bath. Then pretend you are floating around the French Riviera. Don't worry . . . you may be soon. Well, as soon as you are ready to leave your house, at any rate.

BAKING SODA BATH
To Sooth and Smooth Irritated Skin

½ cup or more baking soda

If you're like me, the minute you get crazed over something, your skin goes whack-o. I mean, it's just not fair . . . you can't even get a broken heart without broken-out skin. If you find that your body becomes itchy and irritated when *you* are, try pouring a half cup or more of baking soda into a tub full of water. The properties of the baking soda not only soothe irritated skin, they actually help to soften it too!

SHAKE IT UP, WAKE IT UP BATH

1 tablespoon honey

When you finally decide that you'd like to wake up, run a bath and add the honey. The natural honey will give your skin a lift and leave it feeling smoother.

A FLOWERED FLOAT
Just for the Sweet Smelling Pleasure of It All

1 tablespoon rosemary flowers
1 tablespoon lavender flowers
1 tablespoon of your favorite herbs

Add the ingredients to your bath as it is filling up, and then just sit back and let your mind wander. The bath is the ultimate luxury . . . and a great way to fantasize the day away. Fantasize about what ever you like . . . but *don't* fantasize about *him* . . . fantasize about a lot of revenge . . . like how he will spend the rest of his life regretting that he blew his chance with you . . . especially after he sees what you are about to become!

BUMPY BOTTOM BATH MITT

Believe it or not, one of these days you'll want to have another love affair. They do strike without notice, you know. And when they strike, you suddenly realize that you haven't shaved your legs, you have old lingerie, and you've got a bumpy bottom. Well, the first two are easy enough to get rid of, but the third usually hangs around, so, if you've got a bumpy bottom and nothing seems to get it smoother, try this: Make a mitt by cutting a square of cheesecloth (about five inches square) and filling the center with dry oatmeal. Twist the ends together and secure with a rubber band. Moisten the mitt when you are ready to use it and rub it vigorously over your bottom . . . and any other part that is dry, flaky, or bumpy. The oatmeal acts as an exfoliant (skin slougher) to eliminate impurities.

MORE ON BUMPY BOTTOMS

In addition to the bumpy bottom bath mitt, you can use a gentle peeling agent such as a five percent benzoyl peroxide lotion. Apply the lotion after you've used the mitt described above, or use a loofah when you shower or bathe.

These bumpy dry patches that can appear on your bottom, or sometimes on your arms are actually a thickening of the outermost layer of skin and are caused by the friction of rubbing skin against clothes. To get *your* bottom smooth as a baby's backside, just slough it off, then slather lotion on. And, guess what? You'll get smooth before your next close encounter.

Bonus tip—Hang a three-tiered aluminum vegetable basket (the kind you use to store veggies) on the neck of the shower. Fill each basket with your favorite bath preparations: a loofah mitt, a few homemade oatmeal mitts, and whatever other essentials you simply can't live without in the tub. It's pretty, it's practical, and it's a good way to store all of your bath toys so that you'll be prepared whenever the urge to dip a bit comes your way. I mean you just never know . . . some of my friends take to the tub the way I take to the bed . . . for days on end.

THINGS TO DO IN THE TUB

KARMA CALMER

Obviously, you are having a bad time and relaxing is a bit difficult, now. If this were the sixties, you'd call it bad karma and go out looking for the perfect mantra. But it's the eighties, so you looked instead for the perfect man.

The upshot? Tension! If you can't relax, at least you can untense some of those muscles. Here's how to do that in the tub (or anywhere for that matter).

Tense up all of your facial muscles as tightly as you can. Hold for a few seconds, relax, and repeat two more times. Then do a series of head rolls. Begin with your head on your chest and simply rotate your head to the side, all the way to the back, and round again to the chin-chest position. Do at least five head rolls!

TRESS STRESS: DESTRESS YOUR SCALP TO STOP FALLOUT

If you've noticed that all of this tension you've been going through has caused you to lose a lot of hair, destress your scalp by working on the vasomotor nerves that control the circulation of the scalp. Begin by massaging the neck and shoulders and then work around and across and all over your scalp. Do this several times a day, if you can. It's okay. People expect you to act a bit bizarrely now.

GIVE YOURSELF A FACIAL

A good thing to do on your shameless day off is to give yourself a facial. Here are a few easy, quick, face fixers that you can make up and put on before you take to the tub. (For a complete guide to at-home facials, see the chapter, "Facials without Fuss").

GREEK DIP FOR NORMAL SKIN

½ cucumber
¼ cup plain unflavored yogurt

Greeks use a similar recipe for a delicious dip, you'll use it for deliciously refreshed skin. Here's how: Peel the cucumber by scoring it into one-and-a-half-inch vertical long strips. (So half of the peel remains on.) Then puree the cuke in a blender or food processor. Add the yogurt and stir it up by hand till the mixture is a nice, creamy consistency. Apply the mixture to your face and neck (avoiding eye area).

Now step into the tub, lie back, and relax. When you step out of the tub, remove the facial by splashing on warm water.

MELLOW YELLOW MASK FOR DRY SKIN

1 very ripe mashed banana
½ teaspoon olive oil

Mix the ingredients together and apply to your face, leaving it on for ten minutes. Then just rinse with tepid water till clean. This make-at homer is so filled with moisturizers that it's like a drink for the dries!

AN EGG ON YOUR FACE FOR OILY SKIN

1 egg white
1½ teaspoon lemon juice

Want a blotter for that oily skin? This one works like crazy . . . and leaves your skin tightened and refreshed.

Just beat the egg white till frothy, and mix in the lemon juice. Apply to your face and leave on for twenty minutes. Remove with lukewarm water.

Bonus tip for all facials—To close up pores, always splash on a few handfuls of cold water after you've completely removed your mask.

EXERCISE YOUR FACE . . . AND YOUR BOD . . . IN THE BATH

While you are slathering around in your beauty bath, waiting for your facial to set, do a few quick, easy exercises that will make you feel truly well cared for. (Don't do any exercise if your facial needs to set without movement, of course.) Just think of all the gorgeous—and easy—things you can do for yourself while Mr. Once-Was is fooling around. God, you're going to be gorgeous . . . and won't *he* be sorry . . . the crumb.

FACE FIRMER

Open your mouth and your eyes as wide as possible. Hold for a full five seconds and relax. Do this ten times.

CHIN UP

To firm your chin, put your head back as far as you can go. Then bring your lower lip up as much as you can . . . as though you were trying to touch the tip of your nose. Hold for a count of six. Relax and repeat ten times.

SUPPORT STRUCTURE
To Help Firm Up Breasts

To firm up the muscles that support the breasts (not the breasts themselves), smile as widely as you can (until it becomes a grimace), hold for a count of ten, and release. Repeat five times. This is a good exercise to do not only in the tub, but whenever you remember to do it. You can also apply washcloths soaked in cold, cold, cold water to your breasts to boost circulation.

Bonus breast tip—Never run the hot shower water on your breasts, ever. It increases the chances of breast sag. NOW, go back to bed. You feel great!!!

8 · Sleep Getters: How to Get Some If You Aren't Getting Any

Sleep. It becomes a main-line function when we are feeling depressed, upset, anxious, or even angry. And since this part of the book is devoted to the things you should consider doing while lying in your bed, anyway, let's get down to the big one: SLEEP.

Someone once asked Loretta Young, a woman considered to be one of the world's great beauties, what her secret beauty routine was. She replied, "Sleep. Lots of Sleep." And that is one of the truest things you will read in this whole book.

Restful sleep can make your eyes brighter, your skin clearer, your whole body look better. Lack of restful sleep, on the other hand, can make you look haggard, dissipated and . . . God Forbid . . . Older!

But what happens? Well, when you are upset you will either crave sleep and spend countless hours doing it as a means of escaping reality (and thus not facing the awful problem that lies in wait during waking hours), or you will lie in bed night after night so disturbed and unable to escape reality that sleep hardly ever comes. Frankly, if given the choice, I would definitely opt for the escape route.

As long as you know that it's temporary, it's certainly not harmful. For one thing, you don't really escape reality entirely when you sleep. In fact, for many, sleep brings the answers that the waking mind is too fuddled up with to answer. For example, Robert Lewis Stevenson credited critical scenes in *Dr. Jekyll And Mr. Hyde* to dreams he had while trying to grapple with impossible passages. And speaking of passages, Hannibal claimed his passage across the Alps was an idea that came to *him* during sleep. Now if Hannibal could handle the elephant question during sleep, chances are good that you can get an insight or two into what's disturbing you, too.

But the first thing you've got to do is to get some sleep. So, if sleep is the thing you'd sell your soul for at this point, but can't find any takers, it's important that you try to discover the *real* reason for your "insomnia." Most probably, if you are reading this book, your problem stems from anger over loss. And loss is one of the most common villains in situational insomnia. So, chances are good that when you find the answer to the problem, you will go back to sleeping your regular pattern.

A single problem, however, can occasionally cause a longer bout of insomnia. How? By transferring your current worry to concern about your inability to sleep! The anxiety over not being able to sleep can become intense enough to cause you to lose more sleep than your original worry had. So, remember that you are suffering a temporary loss of sleep caused by your problem; you ARE NOT AN INSOMNIAC. In fact, even if you *think* you aren't getting any sleep, you probably are. For example, some people dream that they are lying awake in bed, because they are afraid that if they fall asleep, they'll lose valuable "think" time. Wrong. As I've said before, sleep can be a time that you can actually work out your problems without stressing yourself.

Think of it this way: Your brain is your computer, and during sleep, you are constantly discarding and dealing with problems in an abstract way that you may not be able to deal effectively with during the day.

Not sleeping, on the other hand, can also increase your depression during waking hours. Even a wonderfully happy person can become depressed if deprived of sleep. And since the two things you need to do right now are to look better and to feel better, you've got to get to sleep. Here's how:

SLEEP . . . SWEET SLEEP: GETTING SOME

The Better Sleep Council has compiled mountains of research on sleep. Here are some of their suggestions.

- *Stay away from caffeine.* And that means all evening . . . maybe all day. The actual peak effect of caffeine takes place from two to four hours after consumption and may last as long as seven hours! That means if you consume a cup of coffee at 8:00 P.M., you may feel the effects at midnight and be energized until 3:00 A.M.! It also can cause you to wake up in the middle of the night. Caffeine stimulates the adrenal glands that produce glucose, and that, as you know, is what gets you moving.

• *Have a drink.* One. A small glass of wine, preferably red, will relax you. More than one will make you pick up a mandolin and start singing old Italian love songs while crying. Seriously, too much wine can disturb your sleep even more.

• *Tap some tryptophan.* L-Tryptophan is an amino acid that is a natural sleep inducer, and unlike sleeping drugs, it will leave no drug hangover. You can bite into some tryptophan by snacking on any of these: cottage cheese, milk, soybeans, chicken, cashews, or turkey.

• *Begin to unwind early in the evening.* If you've a mountain of work to complete, get started early. Don't read anything that is too gripping, scary, or romantic. The first two will tense you up, the third will make you depressed if you're trying to recover from a love affair.

• *Breathe deeply* . . . it can bring on drowsiness, by accumulating carbon dioxide in the body. Here's how: Take very slow, deep breaths in a series of three, exhaling fully after each. After the third, hold your breath as long as you can, and then repeat the series. After five to eight series of three, you'll want to breathe normally and you'll want to sleep!

• *Feel secure.* If you've recently split up with the man who was occupying the other side of your bed, you may be feeling as though you are now fair prey for all of the killers and weirdos in the world. Buy a dog; they're even better protection than a new man, but do whatever you have to do to feel secure. Have new locks installed, put in a smoke alarm, or even get a new unlisted phone number. But feel secure or you'll be awakened by every single noise.

• *Get some exercise.* Yes, yes, I know I promised that I wouldn't force you to go out just now, and I won't. You can exercise at home. Jump rope, run in place, but try to do it in the morning, and don't exhaust yourself and bring on fatigue that can cause lack of sleep.

• *Daydream.* Think about revenge: Plot a good one with you as the star, and Mr. Once-Was as the fool. Remember, if he didn't love you, he's just a jerk . . . probably not a villain. If he *is* a villain, however, the best revenge you can ever have is simply not caring about him. Villains hate that.

• *Take a bath.* Warm—not hot. Baths are the world's most luxuriously wonderful excesses one can have . . . and you've just learned the most excessive ones of all. Pick one out of the previous chapter and then choose your prettiest, silkiest nightie to sleep in when your bath is over.

• *Don't nap between sleeps.* If you can't sleep at night, try not to nap during the day. You won't be as tired at your regular bedtime.

• *Avoid stimulants* and snacking on any foods that will make your digestive system more active. Keep away from diet pills and antidepressants because they can keep you awake forever. It has even been shown that some birth-control pills have caused insomnia. If you suspect that any drug you are taking has interfered with your sleep, consult your doctor and get a replacement pill.

• *Avoid noise.* If the slightest noise is making you crazy (and it can do that when you're feeling down), do everything you can to soundproof your environment. If you live in a big city and are subjected to the street sounds, get a set of ear plugs.

• *Keep it dark.* If your rooms let in too much light, you simply will not sleep as well as in complete darkness. If, however, you feel insecure without "that" man when it's pitch black, you can disregard this tip altogether and keep a small light burning. Being frightened will keep you awake longer than a light will.

• *Love your bed.* Get a whole new set of linens and make it look wonderful and just the opposite of what it looked like when it was occupied by Mr. Once-Was. I personally find that I feel best when I turn my bed into a Camille-like frilly place of repose during periods of recovery. But whatever works best for you is what you should do . . . pleasant dreams!

9 · Assess Your Assets: The Best Tests to Take When You've Taken to Your Bed

Think about this: In a few months you will be over the worst of what you are feeling now. In a few months you will begin to want to go out and meet new men again. In a few months you are also, most importantly, going to look and feel like a whole new lady. You are going to be on your way to becoming a beauty . . . even if you weren't born that way! (And who was?)

And in a few months you are going to be that much more in control of your life than you are right now. But right now, I'm going to insist that you start pampering yourself. That's right, indulging yourself on a day off is only the beginning! You are now about to make that indulgence a permanent part of everything you do. You are about to learn that your happiness comes before everything else. After all, it's your life and if you aren't going to bring happiness and love into it, nobody else will. You must learn that you have to do that yourself.

But right now, just remember that even if you are still feeling crummy and unable to go out and have fun, the least you can do is stay home and have fun plotting your gorgeous revenge.

Let's start out by getting a whole picture of your weak points and strong points. That way, you'll know whether you need to cover up, expose, or pad your account.

No matter what the following tests tell you, you will find a way or two in each of the following chapters to correct what's wrong and build up what's already terrific. I know that you think it's too much effort to do anything right now (besides put one foot in front of the other), but once you start, you'll find that you're not only enjoying yourself, but you're looking better every minute.

Think about the goal you've set for yourself: Isn't it going to make you feel better than you've ever felt when you look better than you've ever looked before? You bet it will! Now, let's get started.

TESTING . . . ONE, TWO, THREE . . . : EVALUATING EVERY PART OF YOU

Let's find out how you stack up. These tests will help you to determine what shape your shape is in, what kind of hair you've got, what kind of skin you're in, and what sort of body you're walking around with.

HAIR-RAISING TESTS FOR TYPE AND TEXTURE

Your hair is your most important beauty accessory. And it's also the place that women run to in times of crisis for immediate gratification. That's because the versatility of it can make the most dramatic changes possible in the shortest amount of time. Let's face it, if you need to lose a couple of hundred pounds, it will take you a bit of time. If you want an immediate change NOW, your hair is the place to start. So, let's start by finding our what you've got to work with.

What's the Texture?

To find out whether you have fine, medium, or coarse hair try this: Gather up a large section of hair and push back the ends. If your hair feels like a baby's brush, it's fine. If it feels like a paintbrush, it's coarse. And if it feels fine at some points and coarse at others, you've got medium-textured hair.

What's the Type?

Begin by washing your hair very thoroughly with a bar of plain soap such as castile or a shampoo that does not contain conditioners. This is to strip away all of the oil and dirt. Let your hair dry naturally and wait a few hours before you look at it very carefully. If it looks limp, but shiny and silky, it's fine/oily. Choose a shampoo that is specially formulated for fine, oily hair. You should also look to see that the shampoo has some sort of body builder in it, to give you volume.

If your hair looks bulky and wiry, it is coarse. Choose a shampoo for dry hair. You need a conditioner, but you don't need more volume, so choose a LIGHT conditioner.

Does your hair look thick and shiny? Lucky You! You have got slightly oily, thick hair. You need a shampoo that contains just a drop of conditioner already in it. All your hair needs is a manager . . . not a boss.

Does it look dull and flyaway even though there's not enough of it to fly very far? Then you've got fine, dry hair. You want a shampoo for dry hair *and* a rich, high-protein conditioner. You *don't* want a shampoo with a conditioner built in because the two conditioners will make you look as though you've glued your hair on.

You might also look into the men's hair care department for a hair thickener. Besides, think about the bonus: Next time a man peeks into your medicine cabinet . . . and they all do . . . he'll think some guy is already leaving his stuff around. It will drive him crazy with curiosity, while you are sitting there with this mane of fabulous hair.

THE SKIN GAME . . . TYPECASTING YOUR FACE

Brown Bagging It

To find out your skin type, try this: Wash your face before going to bed at night. Then, before you tuck in, place several skin-blotting papers or strips of brown paper bag next to your bed. When you awaken in the morning, rub one piece of paper across your forehead, one on your nose, one on either cheek, one across your chin.

Where the paper shows just a tiny bit of shine, your skin is normal, where it shows no shine at all, it's dry, and where it is translucent, or very shiny, it's oily.

CHARTING YOUR CORRECT WEIGHT

Whoever invented those weight charts anyway? Why, for God's sake, did they give you height measurements with shoes on?! Was the world so crazed in the fifties when the charts were invented that the chartmakers thought they'd be brought up in front of the House Un-American Activities Committee for shamelessly weighing people with naked feet? Well, the insurance companies are beginning to change the charts, and have finally come up with a chart based not only on age, but, praise the Lord, bare feet. (The clothes are still on, however.)

Interestingly, the belief now is that the average weight for your height isn't the "ideal" weight. In fact,

YOUR IDEAL WEIGHT*

Height	Age 20 to 29 (lb.)	Age 30 to 39 (lb.)	Age 40 to 49 (lb.)	Age 50 to 59 (lb.)	Age 60 to 69 (lb.)
4 ft. 10 in.	102	106	111	114	117
5 ft. 1 in.	112	115	120	123	126
5 ft. 4 in.	120	123	129	133	135
5 ft. 7 in.	131	135	139	143	145
5 ft. 10 in.	142	148	151	154	155

*In clothing, no shoes.

a person weighing ten percent less than "average" has the best chance for a longer life.

WEIGH TO GO! (A FAT FORMULA TO LIVE BY)

If charts and tape measures aren't enough for you . . . or you just don't feel like getting out of bed right this minute, follow this simple formula to find your ideal weight. You'll notice that the weights differ slightly from the chart, which is done with your clothes on. Start with the height of five feet and 100 pounds. (If you are five feet, that is your ideal weight.) Then add five pounds for each inch over five feet. So, if you are five feet, six inches your ideal weight is 130 pounds. If you've a small body frame, subtract ten percent. If you are large framed, add ten percent. Now, that was easy, wasn't it?

FINDING YOUR FRAME

Are you small, medium, or large framed? Doesn't it make you crazy to look at those "ideal weight charts," never knowing the truth? Well, here's a test that will tell you the truth. You may, however, need a lie-detector test next, because if you are like me, you'll lie about your frame size each time you see a box of Ring Dings.

How in the world do you know whether you are small, medium, or large framed? Try this:

Measure your height to the nearest quarter inch. Next, get a friend to measure around your shoulders with a tape measure. Add your weight to your shoulder circumference. If the total is less than 99, you have a small frame. If it falls between 99.1 and 106, you have a medium frame. If the total is more than 106, your frame is large.

THE SHAPE-YOUR-TUMMY-IS-IN TEST

When you ponder the ultimate questions of the universe, does your mind keep returning to the ultimate question: "Am I really fat?" If you truly are, you already know it, but if you are just starting out, this test will let you know, and hopefully stop you before you ease on down the road any further.

Remember, though, that when you've been rejected, devastated, or feel lonely, you will think of yourself as fat and unattractive no matter what. Here's how to measure up:

Subtract your waist measurement from your height in inches. If the answer is *less* than thirty-six, it's time to get going and get into shape!

Flex Test

Here's a test for flexibility: Bend at the waist and try to touch the floor. You should be able to reach ground level with your fingertips. If you can't you can use some stretching exercises. And now's a great time to start stretching into place. Remember, for great sex, you need great flex.

Sit Up and Take Notice

How strong are you? No, not emotionally . . . physically. (You may not realize it yet, by the way, but you are quite strong emotionally, or you wouldn't be reading this book and you wouldn't be ready to conquer the blahs.)

To test your strength, try sit-ups. If you can do twenty-five or more in one minute, you are okay, kid. If you fall short, you can use some muscle developers, such as pushups and sit-ups.

THE BREAST TEST

Someday you will decide that you'd like to go out again. Someday you will also decide that you'd love to make love again. Well, if you had been with the same man for a long while, chances are good that you aren't sure how a new man will like your body. And for most women, "body" generally means breasts. Do you feel that your breasts just aren't what they once were, or have never been what they once were? Then take this test. It will help you to see probably just how wrong you are. If you find that your breasts really aren't firm enough, get busy during this down time to firm up so that you'll be self-confident . . . not self-conscious during your next daring close encounter. But, most importantly . . . remember that you will never allow yourself to love anyone ever again who doesn't think that you are *already* perfection!!! This test is for *you*—not for the new *him!*

Stand in front of a mirror sans bra. Take an eyebrow pencil and place the blunt end on the nipple and the sharpened end against your forearm in a straight line. Now mark the spot on your arm. Look at where the mark is on your arm. If it is midway between your elbow and shoulder, chances are good that your breasts are firm enough to stand up on their own. If the mark falls below that center point, you should begin doing some of the isometric toners and other exercises that you will find later on in the book. (Yes, they really *do* work!)

10 · Hair-Raisers: A Bunch of Wonderful Things to Do to Your Hair When You're Miserable

WHAT YOUR HAIRSTYLE SAYS ABOUT YOU!

Before we go any further and begin to fix what ails your hair, let's take a look at the way you *wear* your hair. How you wear your hair will give you an insight not only into yourself but also into the way people react to you. And since women who are coming out of a marriage or love affair tend to go first to the hair, let's take a look at how you wear it now, and how you'd like to wear it in the future. Most hairdressers will tell you that when a woman is feeling emotionally upset, she'll come in and demand a whole new style. Now, I don't think that is wrong at all. After all, you want to make some changes, right? But, before you do, think carefully about why you have worn your hair a certain way. Why do you want to change it? Don't do something out of revenge that will backfire on you. Learn to talk to your hairdresser. It's important that this person understand your lifestyle. If you are tight for time, you don't want a style that you're going to have to fuss with every minute, for example.

But what about the way you wear it now? If you've had the same style for years it might mean that you've found a style that's perfect for you. It might even be part of your total look. Many stars like Lauren Bacall and Dolly Parton are instantly recognizable by their hairdos and haven't ever changed the look. But chances are good that you aren't Lauren Bacall or Dolly Parton. An unwillingness to change might mean that you've been clinging to an old style for comfort. Comfort is nice . . . but it sure isn't exciting. And what we want to do now is to shake up your style and your life, a little. Oh, hell . . . a lot!

Do you tease your hair into a helmet for a conehead? Then you are either *very* new wave, or really old hat. If it's old hat, it's definitely time for a change. If it's new wave, be careful! Why? Because men are afraid of hair that doesn't move! Scientific evidence has proved that nine out of ten men shrink back in horror and fear when asked to run their fingers through a beehive!

Seriously, though, stiff, "done," oversprayed, or perfect styles subconsciously tell people that you don't want to be touched. And guess what? They might just stay away! If that sounds like you, try letting loose for one day only just to see how people react to you, and you to them. Write down your experience. Then take the paper out in a few days or weeks, and see if the reaction was good enough to do it again . . . and again.

Or are you a lady who is *always* trying new styles? Then people might think of you as someone with a strong self-identity. But is that so? Do you constantly change because it's fun (and it is) or do you change because you are too insecure to be fifteen seconds behind the trends? If that sounds closer to the truth, why not try something completely different, and go for a classic look once in awhile? You'll be amazed at the different reactions you get from everyone. You'll also be amazed at the different sort of man you attract and that's what this book is all about—change.

Do you wear your hair pulled back into a bun or tight pony tail? Then the first impression you give off is that you are a cool-headed, conservative person . . . the kind of lady who can hold her own. If you like the look, and it's right for you, then go with it. But why not occasionally team your hairstyle with something a little unexpected such as a bunch of gold ribbons that float down your back or a really frilly blouse? It's the sort of trick that makes people (men in particular) think of you in a different light (and gives them fantasies of untying the ribbon to see your cascades of tumbling curls). They will never know that you may have pulled your hair back in a bun to hide the fact that you haven't washed it.

Speaking of cascades of tumbling curls . . . is that your everyday look? If so, you're giving off signals that say you are a soft and feminine woman. That's great for parties, but not so wonderful if you mean business at the office. If you want to move up to the executive suite (your own, not someone else's), then you might try pulling your hair up into a French twist or French braid for the office. Both styles are chic, no-fuss, timeless, and feminine, but in a more businesslike way.

Short, cropped hair, on the other hand, conveys the image of someone who is a no-nonsense type, one who is more concerned with what she is doing than how she may look doing it. But that is not *always* so. Short trendy cuts brushed high on top and tapered short in the back, for example, convey a high-fashion image. Short wash-and-wear cuts convey an image of someone who is more efficient than elaborate. But a great short cut can stand perfectly well on its own . . . it's the cut and the cutter that make *all* the difference. If you have been wearing the same short cut for a long time, try something radically different with it once in awhile. For example, set it wet on sponge rollers, if you normally wear it straight. If you normally wear it curly, slick the sides back and curl or backbrush the top for a ton of volume.

Do you wear bangs? Well, if your hair or bangs cover more of your face than is revealed, you give the impression that you are shy, or just don't have the confidence to face the world straight on. Try snipping them to just below the eyebrows, and curling them up and back for the brand-newest look. That's what I do with mine, and I love it! In fact, since I've discovered this new trick, I think I will keep bangs forever. You can wear them down, back, or curled. And you can let them grow out whenever you want to without looking like a twelve-year-old good girl.

One final word about how you wear your hair. No matter what style you wear, don't wear it too neatly, unless you are going to a black tie dinner. Hair that is too neat says "stay away," for one thing, and makes you look like a Stepford Wife for another. It scares people away because it makes you look unfriendly, untouchable, and untenable. Think not? Take a look at what goes on at the next cocktail party you attend. The woman who is so put together that she looks as if she should be encased in Lucite is never the one who is at the center of the action. It's usually the one whose hair, clothes, and makeup say

61

that she's open and fun. The gorgeous creature who has spent hours getting ready is the one whom everyone usually admires . . . from afar. From a very far.

BREAKING AWAY

How to Find the Right Hairstylist

Now, I know you're thinking that the last thing on earth you need—or want—to do right now is to go to the hairdresser. If you don't want to, you don't have to. This book is not designed to put any pressure on you at all. But I am saying that sometimes what you really need to do is to break away from the past by letting go of a lot of the things that tie you to it. Sometimes, those old, familiar patterns are boring, and sometimes they are just so much a part of your routine that you aren't even aware of whether they are viable for you anymore. So, when you are ready to get out and make a change, maybe you should start with your hairdresser. Here's why:

You want to change, you want to look like a whole new lady (or you will someday soon). You want to feel great about yourself again. You want that crumb to regret that he made you so miserable!! You *want* him to be miserable. (Don't deny it. We're not talking about being altruistic here . . . we're talking about getting you over this time.)

Anyway, one of the best ways to get a new look and a new attitude going is to find a new hairdresser. A new hairdresser will see you in a whole new light. She (or he) will be trying harder to please you because you are a new and potentially regular customer. I say, if you want to get a new look, start with a new hairdresser. But finding a new hairdresser who's right for you is often more difficult than finding the right style. Anyway, it's a good way to go out without too much brain pain. And chances are more than good that you won't run into you-know-who sitting in the next chair. One word of caution: Be careful about the music that they have piped into the shop. I once found myself shamelessly sobbing to a song that "we" used to love to dance to. It wouldn't have been quite as horrifying if I hadn't been getting my hair highlighted at the moment and had tin foil rods sticking out of my head.

Here, then, a bunch of ways to find someone who's right for you (a hairdresser, anyway):

• Next time you see someone with a great short hair cut, stop her and ask for the name of her hairdresser. Don't just be envious that her hair cut is better than yours—find out who does it!! Short hair, incidentally, is a much better indicator of hair-cutting talent than long hair. Long hair is a statement more about the wearer than the cutter.

• When you find a new hairdresser, go in early and watch him or her work. If you feel uncomfortable in the environment, leave! Don't be embarrassed. Blaring music and disco hairdressers make almost everyone uncomfortable! And you are learning now that you needn't ever do anything that will make you uncomfortable again!

• Watch your hairdresser work. Most pros look from the mirror to the client rather than just at the client's head. This gives a hairdresser the whole picture.

• Don't forget that you are *hiring* a hairdresser each time you go in. So act like a boss, not like a slave. Don't let him or her intimidate you . . . you are in a fragile enough state as it is right now. The last thing you need is some pushy hairdresser pushing you around!

• Look in the local papers at the ads and editorials that feature beauty salons and hairstyles. Call the place and ask about the stylist who did the hair in the picture.

• Make sure the stylist consults with you before you are told to change your clothing. It's important for the hairdresser to see how you're dressed. It will tell him something about you . . . namely, what you are comfortable with.

• Finally, get your hair cut in a salon, not a boutique. Beauty shops that also sell clothing and jewelry are more concerned with mark-ups than with hair cuts!

The Cost of Getting Gorgeous

A good cut doesn't come cheaply. But then again, neither does your time. Your time *is* money and you shouldn't spend hours of it maneuvering around a bad haircut. So cut your costs by cutting your hair . . . properly. Here's a breakdown of what hair care at better salons around the country will cost you:

• *Cut*—$25 to $50. Needs to be done every four to six weeks.

• *Color*—Anywhere from $25 on up. Needs to be done every four to six weeks.

• *Highlighting*—A more exacting process is also a more expensive one: $30–$150. Needs to be done every few months, or as often as you wish.

Tips on Tipping

Confused, embarrassed, or just plain stumped when it comes to tipping at your favorite salon? You'll be right on the money if you use the following rules:

- *Haircutter*—10–15% of the total bill. (In larger cities, 20% is sometimes given, although it's not expected.)
- *Hair Colorist*—10–15%
- *Shampoo Person*—$1.00
- *Manicurist (and/or Pedicurist)*—20%
- *Makeup Artist*—20%

And remember, you are not expected to tip the salon owner if she's the one who does your hair. Furthermore, don't feel obligated to tip someone who hasn't done a good job. There's no reason on earth to tip anyone who has made you feel badly, or worse, made you look badly.

Remember, TIPS means: To Insure Preferential Service. If you didn't get it, don't do it. A creative genius who make you cry, gives you green hair, or a Grace Jones haircut deserves only one tip from you: the suggestion that he find a new line of work.

MAKING WAVES: A BUNCH OF QUICKIES TO GET YOUR HAIR SHAPED UP, SHINED UP, SET UP . . . FAST!

Beginning to get antsy sitting around the house feeling awful? Well, that means that very soon you are going to start wanting to get back out there. And if you are now or ever have been depressed and anxious your hair is going to take the brunt of that stress. You might find it thinner, lifeless, and looking as depressed as you feel. Fear not. Help is on the way.

So, if you find that very soon you want to go, you need to go, you'd like to go, but your hair says no, experiment with any or all of the following hair savers. They are fun, they are easy, and they work so quickly that you won't have time to change your mind about going out.

For Hair to Go: Sets to Stay

JET SET

This trick takes a few minutes and lasts for hours. Apply a setting lotion to dry hair, and set it on soft, absorbent sponge rollers, or old-fashioned cloth curlers (the kind with the wire inside). Grab a section of hair, twist it around the roller, secure or bend into place. Then take your blower and blow the set dry. Unwrap the rollers and finger comb into place. Spritz with a soft hair spray and go.

SET THAT SET TO HOLD THAT STYLE

You still aren't feeling great, but you know that you still want to look good. God knows you don't want to run into *him* (or someone even more interesting) with your hair set. So, when you've errands to run, but don't want to lose your set, or your dignity, by going out with curlers, try this trick: Just remove the curlers, shake your head, and spray your hair with hair spray. Don't brush it out. If your hair is short, just very lightly finger comb it to remove the roller ridges. If it's long, put it up in a bun, and spray it again. This will hold your set until you are ready to style your hair.

HEAD SET

This one from the hair pros at Gillette. Wash your hair and spray it with hair spray while it is still wet. Let it dry and *then* set it on rollers. After you remove the rollers, spray again before you lightly finger comb or brush out. What will you have? Lots of volume and lots of curl, that's what. Now, how can you look at that gorgeous head of curls and feel dumpy?

TITLE WAVES
For a Rich-Girl Head of Deep, Controlled Waves

Spray wet hair with hair spray, or styling lotion, then simply pick up small sections of hair, twist tightly into curls around forehead, and secure each in place with a decorative/holding type of comb. Spray once more, let it dry, and brush out lightly.

HOT HEAD
A Quick Pro Set That Lasts

Finger dry wet hair, then curl a section of hair around a pencil, slip the pencil out, and wrap the curl in a precut rectangle of aluminum foil. Turn the ends to secure. Then sit under a hair dryer for about ten minutes or so. Allow your hair to cool before lightly brushing out.

SCULPT TRESS

Ready to sculpt your hair into shape? Apply setting lotion or hair spray to very damp hair. Use your fingers to separate and lift the strands, creating air pockets. Then softly shape into place with a blower brush, or a brush and blower. You are actually "sculpting" the waves by pushing them into shapes. Let your hair dry naturally.

SET-TO-STAY SETTING LOTION

Even if you're not ready to go out and play, you can stay home and play with different looks. This easy, inexpensive make-at-homer will turn out to be a must-do when you *are* ready, however.

Simply mix together 1 part of grapefruit juice with three parts of water. Apply to semidry hair before you set it, and then forget it. There's nothing else to do.

CREATE A CURLER

Want a head of curls, but you don't even *own* a curler? Don't panic. Let's be honest, *no one* has curlers anymore. A roller or two and several blow dryers, yes, but curlers? Well, curlers are making a return engagement, and can give you a head of curls or waves in no time flat. If you need some curlers—quickly—make your own. Here's how:

Yarn Ties

Cut several pieces of yarn into five-inch long strands. Fold the pieces in half so that it resembles a hairpin. Wind a one-inch section of hair around the bottom half of the "pin" and roll up toward your scalp. Tie the two ends together. Repeat all over your head.

Cut aluminum foil into four-inch-long lengths. Twist the foil to resemble rods. Use the same procedure as mentioned above and twist the two ends together to secure.

And remember, you can get the same effect by using rags, pipe cleaners, even paper toweling (but not on wet hair, of course).

MORE HOME TIPS

Bang Boom

Bangs are back (and boy, can they change your look!), especially layered bangs, which can give you an elegant pompadour (very *au courant*) when brushed back, or a younger more innocent look when brushed forward. Ask your hairdresser about layering the top of your hair into bangs. If he looks confused, and you suspect that he doesn't know what you are talking about, run away. Don't let him touch you. You might end up looking like Imogene Coca or Rod Stewart. And *that* you don't need now.

Here's how to shape 'em, no matter what shape they take:

• *Pompadour*—Spray your hair, brush bangs back, and style. Or try gentle teasing, which will help to train them to stand back and high.

• *Forehead Fringe*—To create full where flat used to be, wrap your bangs around your finger, and then spray with hair spray. Or place a round brush under your wet bangs at the hairline. Don't wrap the hair around it, just rest it there. Then gently blow dry on a medium setting.

• *Punk Spunk*—Use hair-setting gels to get your bangs to: stand up, lay flat, slick back, stick out, frizz up, and head in every direction at once. Swell gels are Tenax and Dippity-Do. If you're still depressed and can't bear the thought of walking to the drug store, call instead. Who knows, they may deliver.

Mane Line Shine:
Bright Ideas and Quick Tricks to Shine up Every Kind of Hair

GETTING INTO CONDITION

RUM TOP . . .
To Shine Up Even the Dullest Hair

Two egg yolks
One jigger of rum

Ready to let rum go to your head? Beat together two egg yolks with the rum. Smooth it on your hair and wrap your head in a warm towel or even in cotton batting. Leave it on for half an hour, and then rinse and rinse again, with cool water.

One more clue—It's always a good idea to use a cool rinse. It smooths down the hair shafts, which reflect the light and bring out the shine. In this case, it's necessary. (You wouldn't want the egg to forget its place and poach on your head.)

GOODBYE DRY
Moisterizer for Dry Hair

2 tablespoons warmed olive oil
1 egg yolk

Apply the mixture to your hair and scalp. Massage in well, and let it sit for about thirty minutes. Then shampoo as usual and rinse with cool water.

COMING CLEAN: GRIME FIGHTERS FOR HAIR

AWESOME AVOCADO SHAMPOO
For Dry, Dull Hair

½ ripe mashed avocado
½ cup nondetergent shampoo
½ cup water

If you want to turn the lights on in even the dullest, splittiest, crummiest hair, start with an avocado and go from there!

Just blend the ingredients together in your blender. Wet your hair and apply the avocado mixture. Massage it well into hair and scalp. Work up as rich a lather as you can. Rinse and rinse and rinse until the hair feels clean. If you still feel that your hair is a bit sticky, use a drop of regular shampoo. Towel dry, style, and fall in love with your hair.

CLEAN SHEEN

No time to wash your hair, or not in the mood? Sprinkle your hair brush with baby powder and then brush, brush, brush to remove excess oil and yuk.

RUM RAISING EGG SHAMPOO
To Build Up Body

1 egg yolk
1 jigger dark rum
Shampoo

Mix the ingredients and use the mixture to wash your hair. Rinse well with cool water. You'll be surprised to see shiny, healthy where stringy, boring used to be.

OIL BLOTTER SHAMPOO
For Hair with an Oil Glut

½ to 1 teaspoon baking soda

If your oily hair shampoo is just not doing the job, raise a stir by stirring in a bit of baking soda. Simply premeasure the amount of shampoo you normally would use for two rinses. Mix in the baking soda and shampoo in the normal manner for more mannerly hair.

PERMANENT SOLUTIONS: HOW TO HOME PERM LIKE A PRO

Remember which twin has the Toni? How could you ever forget? Well, home perms have come a long way since the days when countless mothers spent countless hours torturing countless daughters with stinging home permanents, which often resulted in the much sought-after frizzies. Home perms *had* to come a long way, or the companies would have gone out of business the second we, the tortured masses, grew old enough to take our hair into our own hands.

Well, while you are taking your life into your own hands, do the same with your hair. A home perm is a great thing to do on Saturday night. It keeps you from feeling sorry for yourself! In fact, call up a couple of women friends and you can do each other's hair, drink beer, and commiserate over a pizza and a perm.

Home perms now can give you anything you want—lots of body, lots of curls, or just soft waves. The choice is yours. And the processes have become so simplified and so varied that you are sure to be able to find just what you need, and get just what you want. The built-in extra of a good perm? Freedom! Well, at least the freedom from fussing and fixing your hair every two seconds.

The Waves You Crave . . . Tips and Tricks

To make sure you get just the results you want, follow these tips from the makers of "Rave" Home Perms, and perm like a pro . . . without leaving home.

Before you begin:

- *Select the right perm.* Look for one specially formulated for your hair type. If your hair has been colored or previously permed, look for specific perms, or perms with specific instructions for color-treated or damaged hair.
- *Read, read, and reread instructions.* Never improvise or you might end up with a lot of frizz and very little hair. Remember, if the directions specify plastic curling rods, don't ever use metal!
- *Get organized.* Assemble everything you need in a

work space that has been cleared for this purpose.

- *Know the look you want before you begin.* Study the package pictures and directions and follow them to the letter. The last thing you want is a surprise.
- *Shampoo your hair.* Lotion penetrates *best* on freshly shampooed, damp hair.
- *Trim the splits.* Have all split and dead ends cut off before you attempt to perm.
- *Remove all jewelry and eyeglasses.*
- *Don't even buy a perm kit if your hair has been hennaed.*
- *Enlist a friend if it's your first time.*

TEST YOUR TRESSES

"Try on" your perm by doing two test curls. This is not only advisable, but necessary if your hair is damaged or color treated.

Here's how: Select two sections for test curls. They should be in the most damaged part of your hair to insure the most drastic results. Follow the directions for regular perming, except that waving lotion should be applied after the test curls are already rolled up. At the time specified on the package, unwind the test curls and check the results. If the hair feels gummy and sticky, it is not in good condition and you must not perm the rest of your hair. Both curls should be rinsed immediately, neutralized, and rinsed again.

If, however, your hair is not sticky or gummy, unwind the curl halfway and push it up toward the scalp. If it forms a soft S curve, your test curl is "done." If it doesn't form a good S, rewind and recheck every few minutes. When you've reached the right degree of curling, unwind the test curls and rinse and complete according to directions. This test-curl time will also tell you how much time you should leave the waving lotion on the rest of your hair.

If you've passed the test curl so far, let the neutral-ized and rinsed curls dry. They should feel silky and be free of all color distortion and breakage. If everything has checked out, you can proceed and perm the rest of your hair.

AS YOU WORK

- For a smooth, sleek look, part off a strand of hair as wide as the curler and about three quarters of an inch deep. Comb and roll thoroughly, but not too tightly. Use small curlers around the neckline, and large and medium curlers for the rest of the hair. For curly tops, make the strand one-half inch deep and use the small plastic curlers all over the head.
- Keep the ends of your hair flat inside the end papers to avoid the dreaded crimp.
- Spray hair with water as you work if it begins to dry.
- Roll the right amount of hair on each curler. Too much hair on a single curler will diminish the amount of wave you get.
- Don't use small curlers where your hair is thin or very short.
- Be sure, as you work, to keep a close check on the time while using waving lotion and neutralizer. A few minutes' difference can mean a world of difference to your hair.

AFTER YOU'RE DONE

- Discard all perm solution and neutralizer. These *cannot* be stored.
- Wait at least forty-eight hours before you sham-poo to set that set and insure that your perm is permanent.

- If you want a curly look, set your freshly permed hair on soft small absorbent rollers. If you want a more relaxed *au natural* style, let your hair dry naturally. If you want a smooth, sleek style, blow dry your permed hair.
- If you color your hair, wait for at least two to three weeks before you attempt to color it again. It's best to check with your hairdresser before you attempt to color your permed hair, however.
- Your hair is more susceptible to damage now, so look for special gentle shampoos and conditioners. Always use a wide-toothed comb to detangle.
- Don't hold a blow dryer too close when drying hair.
- Cover hair while swimming, sunning, or skiing. Trust me. You *will* have enough energy to roam from home just for the fun of it again! (And yes, you will go swimming and skiing again . . . unless of course, you've never gone before . . . in which case, give it a try!)

COLOR YOUR WORLD . . . OR AT LEAST YOUR HAIR

When we think of changes . . . BIG changes . . . the first thing we think about is hair color. Boy, can that change you in a flash. And, unlike cutting your hair, which is what you might want to resort to immediately after a break-up, coloring your hair is reversible (or at least returnable).

Hair is immediate. You don't have to wait to look completely different. Sometimes, the change is *just* the thing you need. Sometimes, however, it is an overreaction to an unhappy situation and you end up more unhappy than before.

But make no mistake about it. I think that everyone who would like to, or needs to, should do it. A new or a renewed hair color can make you feel younger, sexier, more alive than before you did it. Who actually needs to? Anyone who is prematurely gray, anyone who has ever thought that life might be better as a redhead, anyone whose hair is light brown blah, dark dull, or salt and pepper. Yes, yes, I know everyone is always saying how attractive salt and pepper and prematurely gray hair is. Attractive is not gorgeous and is not the same as sexy.

Salt-and-pepper attractive is for Mrs. Father Knows Best and pot weavers who live in communes (that haven't been told the war is over). Aside from women who are deliberately trying to look sexless, I can't think why anyone would add years to their looks with gray and dull hair. Now, don't start screaming and saying that I'm not a feminist (let's call me an individualist). I just happen to think that most gray is aging. There are, of course, exceptions. For example, I have a friend who's in her forties with the most gorgeous short-cropped gray hair ever. But she's not thirty and she's not adding years to her look; she's looking gorgeously her own age. (Although I did notice that she's recently put a blonde rinse in her hair and added a twenty-eight-year-old man to her life.)

Well, anyway, right now over one third of all American women color their hair and the majority are over thirty-five and are doing so to cover gray. So go out and do it. You'll feel ten years younger.

When You Go It Alone . . . Make Sure You're in Good Company: Hair Coloring at Home

Okay, so you've decided that you want to change your hair color, and you want to change it NOW. First, you should know about all of the options that are available to you. For example, you may want to start with a temporary rinse, to "try on" the color before you actually commit yourself to this major change. Or you may decide that you only want to cover gray, or add highlights. So be sure you know exactly what you want and how long you want it to last before you color your hair. The last thing you need now is to end up with orange hair, a red face, *and* a broken heart.

So let's take the guess work—and the fear—out of going it alone by deciding how each procedure works and how each will fit into your lifestyle. For example, a two-step blonding process needs constant attention. Do you have the time? A henna, on the other hand, can give you highlights and *shouldn't* be done more than every few months. But the change you get is not that dramatic. Is that what you want? Herewith, truth and the consequences:

• *Semipermanent Color.* Shampoo-in product that doesn't contain peroxide. This sort of product may be the best way to go at first, because it will cover gray, change your color somewhat, and will give you a lift without a risk. The effect lasts through five to six washings. It's best to start out with a color slightly lighter (but no more than two shades) than your natural color, to get the hang of it. *Time requirement:* half an hour or so every few weeks. You might want to try *Clairol's Color Renewal System,* or a similar product.

• *Permanent Color.* What you see is not always what you get. Permanent color penetrates the innermost cortex of the hair and affects natural color. You can probably go one or two shades lighter and one shade darker without making a drastic change that you don't want to live with. If you are coloring your hair for the very first time, consult the side panels on the boxes carefully to be sure that your color and the color that you are shooting for are not only possible, but sane. Permanent color takes a bit longer, as you must section and "paint" the hair, but it also lasts much longer. Like, forever. *Time requirement:* retouch *only the roots* every five to six weeks. *Nice 'N Easy*®, Preference®, Excellence® and *Clairesse*® are good coloring agents.

• *Two-Step Blonding.* This process takes much more of a commitment, but also gives you the most dramatic of all changes. This is the true glamour-girl blonde. As the name implies, two-step blonding requires two processes: one to lighten the hair and one to color it the shade you want. *Time requirement:* three to four hours ONCE A MONTH. If you don't do it religiously, you will end up with stripes. You must be prepared to keep it up once you start it up.

• *Rinse.* For fun color. This sort of product lasts only until your next shampoo, but it can let you know what your hair would look like blacker, browner, or redder. This can also cover gray when you have to hide it immediately. *Time requirement:* There is no commitment to a rinse. You can do it every time you shampoo or never again. *Nestlé Rinses* are a good bet.

• *Frosting.* This kind of process is for you if you

want dramatic rather than subtle blonde highlights. The blonde color is supposed to *contrast* with your natural hair shade. The look here is dramatic . . . not natural, and it seems to work best on layered hair. *Time requirement:* The commitment is only about twice a year. But know what you want before you frost your hair.

- *Highlighting*
    - HAIRPAINTING. For naturally medium-brown and lighter hair only. This is the very natural-looking way to go lighter without making a big deal about it. You can add highlights that look just as if the sun is shining on your hair or you can be bolder and look as if you've truly lightened your hair. *Time requirement:* There is actually *no* requirement because the random blonde strands blend in with your own hair. The choice of whether you choose to "paint" your hair again or not is yours. *Quiet Touch Hairpainting* Brush-On Highlights are good products.
    - HENNA. A method of "staining" the hair that is as ancient as it is modern. Henna is made from plant roots and stems, and is a nontoxic natural vegetable coloring. Hennas are available in black, brown, red, and neutral shades. Hennas can be used to permanently add body, dramatic sheen, and color to the hair. You cannot use henna to lighten your hair, however. The advantages of using henna? For one, there usually is not a visible "root line," because the color tends to fade somewhat. It is also fairly easy to do at home without making a major monthly commitment. In fact, it isn't even *safe* to do it every month. Once every few months

is the *max*. More than that will dry your hair out unmercifully. Hennas are permanent and you should not color with regular dyes afterwards. You should not use henna if you hair is more than fifteen percent gray, if you have a perm, or have used hair dyes that are still on the hair. Personally, I've changed my opinion on henna and don't recommend it. I'd rather you try one of the new cellophane colors instead.

If henna *is* the way you choose to go, I do suggest that you choose a color as close to your own as possible, because henna is not like marriage . . . it *does* last forever. In fact, it's easier to get rid of a husband than it is to get rid of a henna. And if you choose the wrong color, you can't divorce it . . . you're stuck with it.

To keep your henna pack as healthy as possible, add an egg or two as you are mixing it up. You can also add the following ingredients to your henna and egg mixture for even more intense color.

FOR BLACKER BLACK—A COIF OF ESPRESSO

Use a cup of black coffee or espresso instead of plain hot water for dramatic black highlights.

BRIGHTER BROWN—TEA-FOR-TWO EGGS

Use the water from tea plus two eggs with your henna.

RIGHTING WRONGS

A quick tip from the Andreas Too Hair Salon in New York: If you've overdone your scalp when you've colored your hair, soothe it by dissolving two Alka Selt-zer® tablets in eight ounces of warm water. Don't drink it! Apply it to your hair, let it sit for thirty minutes, and then wash. Do this two times a week to soothe scalp and help hair.

DO'S AND DONT'S FOR AT-HOME HAIR COLORING

If you'd like to cover that gray or just change your hair color, keep these tips in mind.

- If you are a mature woman, keep the color light, even if your natural color was very dark. A dark frame around your face tends to emphasize skin lines and wrinkles, while a light color tends to make them appear softer.
- Don't shampoo before coloring your hair. It can contribute to scalp sensitivity.
- Avoid harsh brushing or scratching your scalp on the day you color your hair. A scratched scalp, or an agitated one can make you see red no matter what color you apply.
- To avoid skin "staining," coat your hairline, tops of ears, and back of your neck with petroleum jelly before you begin.
- Clear out your "work" area, so that you won't dye your towels, toothbrush, and whatever else may be around, if the haircoloring splatters.
- Avoid too much sun exposure after you've colored your hair. It can turn your dark dazzle to dull, and your blonde to brass. It can dry it out, no matter what the color.
- Avoid extremes, especially now. If you are going

lighter, or darker, select a color not more than three shades away from what you've already got. For example, if you are going to be lightening your hair, go from a dark shade to a medium shade, or from a medium shade to a light shade. It will look more natural, and you'll feel more believable, than if you go from a very dark shade to a very light one.

• If you are heavily grayed and want to go for blonde, choose a darker blonde tone, because it will deposit more color on the gray hair than a lighter shade will. And the end result will be a lovely, tawny color.

• Enlist the aid of a friend, especially if this is your first time. You won't be able to reach the back hairs as easily as the front and you could make a mistake, and then get depressed.

• Keep it in great condition. Use a good conditioner every time you shampoo, and treat yourself to a deep conditioning at least once a month to keep the color shining. Remember, hair that is colored simply does not behave the same as untreated hair. No matter how wonderful the product, you will need extra care to keep hair up to par.

Bonus tip—some great commercial conditioners are Nexxus, Nucleic A, Kolestral, and Condition from Clairol.

QUICK COLOR

Does your hair look as boring as you feel right now? Then take a minute to add some glimmer, with any of these do-at-homers. These make-at-home rinses will perk up your hair . . . and your mood . . . in minutes. And

guess what? You may not even have to go to the store
. . . you probably have the ingredients sitting right there
in your house right now. These are very temporary rinses
and will wash out next time you shampoo. Have fun, try
a few.

GIL FERRAR'S BLACK LIGHTS
For Brunettes Only

½ ounce shampoo
10 drops Gentian Violet
1 overripened mashed avocado
rubber gloves
plastic wrap

Want to turn the lights back on in your brunette hair?
Then simply mix the first three ingredients together.
Shampoo as usual and apply the mixture (concentrating
especially on the ends of your hair). Cover your head in
plastic wrap and let the mixture do its stuff for 30 minutes. Then rinse thoroughly.

OR MORE . . .

Black and brunette hair will look brighter with either of
the following rinses. All you need do to get shined up is
shampoo your hair and apply the *cooled* mixture. Let it sit
for a few minutes, then rinse it out.

- To darken it, perk a pot of coffee!
- To sparkle it, brew a pot of tea (orange pekoe
works well).

BLONDE BRIGHTS

To lighten it, comb undiluted lemon juice through it and sit in the sun for half an hour, then rinse out. Or try a product like *Sun In* or *Summer Blond* . . . they work like a dream.

To brighten it, rinse with a brew of two cups of cooled camomile tea.

Now, you've got all the tricks and you've no excuse not to brighten up your hair . . . and yes . . . your life!

Remember, at some point too much pain shows. And unless you start to do something positive about it you'll be unhappy longer than you need to. So, go ahead: Wash that gray—and that man—right out of your hair.

BLACK AND BLUE? HAIR CARE FOR BLACK WOMEN

Are you black and blue because your hairdo, among other things, won't do? Since black hair is so very fragile, anything you do to it can make it prone to breakage. If you've got a broken heart, you don't need anything else broken! So let's not forget about tress stress. As you read this chapter, you'll probably be amazed to see just what sorts of everyday things—such as the way you sleep—can break your hair.

For the answers, and the questions, we went right to the source: Michael Weeks, creator of the Michael Weeks' Hair Care System for Black Hair.

But first, let's get down to basics:

Basic Black Backgrounder

The tight natural curl of black hair comes from hair shafts that are flat and oblong in shape. (This tight curl to the hair, incidentally, evolved to keep the head cool while allowing the neck to perspire in hot climates.) Hair shafts shaped this way cause light to be diffused when it hits the hair, making it look dull. So it's important that you add sheen.

Fragile! Handle with Care

Dry scalp is a common black hair problem, so it's best to use a gentle shampoo, one especially formulated for black hair. Follow up with a good conditioner *always*. And, if possible, stay away from blow dryers. They can be harsh when used often. Choose, if you can, a style that will allow your hair to dry naturally. When you want to switch to sleek curves occasionally, be sure to precondition with a conditioner that is specially formulated for heat-treated hair!

How You Wash Your Face May Be Ruining Your Hair

Michael Weeks has discovered that many "receding" hairline problems are caused by cleansing-product residue (soaps, face creams), which remains on the hairlines, causing hair to break off. This is especially true for permed or relaxed hair. So always take special care to rinse your hairline after every face cleansing. You might also try wrapping a scarf around the hair to prevent soap from touching your hair at all.

You may begin to see the hair that you thought was receding begin reseeding!

Bedding Down

Bedding down, too, can be disastrous . . . at least to your hair. So, be extremely cautious about the type of blankets you use. Blankets made with synthetic or acrylic fibers tend to catch onto the hair strand, pulling the hair out from the follicle, which adds to hair breakage. The key to your good locks? Satin or cotton sheets (and pillow slips) between the blanket and you.

What's Hot and How to Get It

Want to get the latest look? Then relax and stop relaxing your hair. Try a California Curl or Jheri Curl, which uses perming techniques, although the process is not similar. Your hair is set on very large rollers, which puts curl in and takes tightness out. The newest way to wear it is blunt cut and chin length. If you prefer it shorter, go one step back and cut it off to about one inch around the entire head.

Braid It

Braiding, too, is back with heavy corn rows and long extensions trailing down the back. For added fun, try the newest extensions, which come in pink, green fuchsia, and even purple.

The final hot look? Long, long agros with very short cropped tops.

What's Not Hot?

Full-blown afros, overstraightened hair, and pushing your hair around into unnatural lines.

11 · Face Savers

THE SKIN YOU'RE IN . . . AND WHAT TO DO ABOUT IT

How much do you know about the skin you're in? Well, the one thing that you probably know for sure . . . at least now . . . is that when you are upset and crazy, so is your skin. And you probably realize that all of those clichés about skin do in fact have some basis in fact . . . as do most clichés.

For example, what about the one that says when you "overreact" you're "thin skinned"? (And when you don't "overreact" you have a "thick skin"?) Hmm, it seems that you just can't win! Well, the truth is, when you are in turmoil, so, generally, is your skin. And now, since you are just lying around anyway, it's a good time to learn the facts, just the facts, about that skin you're in.

Did you know that the skin is the largest organ of the body, and that your skin weighs almost one sixth of your total body weight? And although the amount varies with the size of your body, many people have enough skin to make a nine-by-twelve-foot rug, which would weigh about eight pounds!

If you've ever been accused of having a thick skin, as we've already mentioned, it might also interest you to know that you'll find the thickest skin on your back, but the most resilient on the palms of your hands and the soles of your feet. The thinnest? On your eyelids. On the average, your body skin is a mere 1.2 millimeters in thickness (about the thickness of four sheets of notebook paper), but it drops to only about .5 millimeters on the eyelids! (That's about half as thick as it is elsewhere.)

As you grow from child to adult, your body weight increases approximately twenty times, but your skin area only seven times. This gives you some idea of the amount of stress naturally placed on the skin . . . not to mention those eyelids!

But what does the skin do aside from saving you the embarrassment of walking around with your liver showing? Well, it's quite interesting actually, because in addition to keeping you together, it retains body fluids, regulates body temperature, and is the body's first line of defense against bacteria and environment.

The skin on your hands? It is sometimes the most telling skin of all . . . at least to your doctor. No, that doesn't mean that he can tell from your chapped hands that you've pulled a Scarlet O'Hara and are now wearing the drapes for a dress. (But then again, in this day and age, it would be nearly impossible to make a dress from drapes. Can you imagine trying to get a belt to fit snugly around vertical blinds?)

Anyway, back to your hands. Yellow palms? It might mean that you have a high level of fat in your blood. Reddening palms? Have you missed a period lately? Red palms are sometimes a first sign of pregnancy. Do you have cold hands (but a warm heart)? An icy grip may indicate that your blood vessels are constricted, which in turn may mean that you're smoking too much.

So hold out your hands . . . examine them closely . . . for the health of it (and you).

Reverting to Type

You already know what type of skin you have (dry, normal, oily), but you might not know that your skin can change and become any one of these at different times, at different ages, and with different emotional states of mind. So you should do the skin type test described in Chapter 9, as often as necessary so that you can change your skin regimen whenever your skin type changes. For example, if you've once had oily skin but now have dry, you may be wrecking it completely, if you are still using drying astringents, lotions, and potions. Got it? Good! Now, here's a basic rundown of what each type of skin is like and what it responds to best.

DRY SKIN: THE WATER SHORTAGE

Dry skin lacks oil, right? Not always. What dry skin usually lacks, according to Dr. Stephen H. Mandy, Associate Professor of Dermatology at the University of Miami Medical School, is water! Water, the component that makes up most of your body, can be sorely lacking in your skin. And the environmentally controlled, hermetically sealed "ideal" environments that we live and work in can make your dry skin that much drier.

Why? Because the heating and air-conditioning systems in homes and offices, which blissfully keep your hair from frizzing, won't keep your skin from drying. You (and I), dear heart, are living in dry, dry air. Think not? Then just take a look at how a long cold winter affects your wood furniture and your plants. All of that dry air being forced into your rooms is also being forced into your skin. And your skin, like your furniture, suffers from surface moisture evaporation.

What to Do?

First you've got to hydrate your skin . . . put back some of the moisture that it's lost. You must also set up a safe barrier between your skin and the environment. A good moisturizer can do that. Basically, there are two types of moisturizers. They are emollients and humectants. An emollient contains necessary lubricants and traps water in the skin. A humectant actually draws the moisture to your skin. Both work, if you use them correctly. To get the most from your moisturizer, apply your moisturizer *over* your predampened skin. Keep a spray can of mineral water handy and spray your face gently before you moisturize it. It's also a good idea to keep a spray can at work and spritz your face several times a day to replenish your thirsty skin. (Evian Brumisateur Atomizer is a terrific one, which you can buy prepackaged.)

Other Ways to Fight the Water Shortage

• If you have a humidifier, use it. It can add the needed moisture to the air. If you don't have a humidifier, then place flat pans of water on the radiator, which can also help humidify the air a bit.

• For all-over body dryness, your bath, according to many experts is your ticket to moister skin. First, cool off your bathwater. Excessively hot water just causes the surface moisture to evaporate, which in turn causes your skin to become even drier. For a slick trick, soak in a bath of plain water for about fifteen minutes. Your skin will have absorbed just the amount of water it needs in that amount of time. Then add your bath oil and soak for five minutes more. The oil will act as a seal on your skin, trapping in the water that your skin has just absorbed.

• Dr. Jean-Claude Bystryn, Associate Professor of Dermatology at the New York University School of Medicine, reminds all of his dry-skin patients that, as we get older, the sebaceous (oil) glands don't function as efficiently as they once did. And that is especially true for the lower legs. If you've no time to lie around in the bath, try Dr. Bystryn's Rx: Step out of the shower and wipe excess moisture off with your hands. *Then* apply your bath oil over your still-damp skin. Step back carefully into the shower for a few seconds to degrease. Step out and dry gently with a soft towel. If you rub too hard, you'll undo all of the moisturizing!

Bonus tip—You can make your own face spritzer by sterilizing a spray bottle and filling it with *mineral water*. All you need do is clean and sterilize the bottle every so often to keep everything clean and fresh. Another good trick is to keep your mister in the fridge. The cool mist feels wonderful!

OILY SKIN AND ACNE: IT'S NOT JUST GREASY KID STUFF

If you have oily skin and are emotionally upset . . . it will show on your skin. If you have oily skin, your sebaceous glands are simply overproducing. That is, of course, a simple way of rounding up a whole complicated series of events, which takes place internally. But oily skin doesn't develop dry skin lines as easily and can keep younger-looking longer. But, of course, nothing is free, so the price you may pay for younger-looking skin, is a "young" person's condition: acne.

If you were ever tortured with acne as a kid, the one thing you knew for sure was that eventually you'd grow up and outgrow your acne. Acne, we were taught, was an affliction that happened to teenagers, and especially to teenagers who deprived themselves of sex while gorging on chocolate bars. This sort of magical thinking also had us looking forward to the age of consent when we would be able to drink, vote, have sex, and clear skin.

Well, we know for sure that the voting and drinking didn't do a whole lot for the skin, but what about the sex? Sorry, guys. Sex, whether there is too much (is that ever a possibility?), or not enough (always a possibility), has nothing to do with skin. (Unless, of course, sex, or the lack of it, makes you so nervous that you break out from the anxiety of it all.)

Well, maybe you are one of the lucky ones whose acne did disappear when it was supposed to. But maybe, just maybe, you weren't quite so lucky. Or perhaps your acne is now making a return engagement after an absence of many years. Does that mean that the existing literature available all of these years is a crock of beans? Is acne *not* just the affliction of adolescence? The answer is, of course, a qualified maybe.

Even though acne is *usually* most active during puberty and adolescence when the hormones are in flux, acne can become reactivated in later life, or it can continue without stop right throughout your adult life.

The reasons, according to Dr. Steven R. Kohn, Assistant Clinical Professor of Dermatology at New York City's Columbia University College of Physicians and Surgeons and Chief of Dermatology at the Hackensack Medical Center in New Jersey, may be vast . . . and varied. The chief suspects are unresolved stress situations, cosmetic misuse, hormonal imbalances, adrenal or liver problems, even undetected ovarian tumors.

So, if you do develop acne as an adult, it is vitally important that you get yourself to a good dermatologist as quickly as possible. And a good dermatologist is one who is not only interested in treating the existing condition, but who is also interested in finding out the *cause* of the existing condition.

But since you are reading this book, you probably are suffering from the number one reason listed above —unresolved stress. So try to calm down to help your skin calm down!

Adult Acne . . . in All Its Forms

Not all acne is the same kind. For example, in recent years, doctors have noticed a whole new form of acne that has begun to appear on the faces of women past puberty and often past menopause! Of course, stress as we've mentioned, can cause an acne eruption at any point because stress actually influences hormonal output, which, in turn, causes an enlargement of the oil glands, which in turn causes acne.

But the most common form of adult acne is self-inflicted: *Acne Cosmetica*. As the name implies, this type of acne is caused by cosmetics. The primary villains are oil-based moisturizers and makeups. These oily cosmetics seep into the pores and hair follicles, clogging them with excess oil. The backed-up oil then produces an acne lesion. Dr. Zenona W. Mally, Assistant Clinical Professor of Dermatology at the Georgetown University Medical School, even advises against the use of moisturizers for all but the driest skins. If you are acne prone and still want to use one, she advises it on the dry areas of your face only. And only use cosmetics and moisturizers that have a water base. Never use any oil-based product if you have oily skin or acne.

Yet another form of acne you can develop as an adult is chin acne. Most of the time chin acne is simply caused by leaning your chin on your hand constantly (which incidentally is something you do more when you are unhappy). The irritation from the constant pressure can cause a breakout.

But, strange as it sounds, chin acne can also be caused by fluoride toothpaste. You may notice that some toothpaste escapes and dribbles down your chin as you are brushing your teeth. Chances are that, instead of rewashing the area, you just wipe it with a towel. Well, the residual fluoride can remain on your skin, causing an acne eruption. So, if it's chin acne you've developed, stop leaning on your chin, and stop using fluoride pastes. In fact, studies have shown that it isn't even necessary for adults to use fluoride, since the preadult years are the cavity-prone ones.

Clean It Up, Clear It Up

Your first step, as we mentioned earlier, is to see a good dermatologist when you feel that you can no longer handle your problem yourself. When you are under stress, the worst thing that can happen to you is that your skin becomes a mess. It makes you fretful, shy, and uncomfortable. (As you know, the only other thing that can make you more self-conscious than suddenly bad skin is suddenly huge thighs.)

The treatments currently in use are wonderful because they reflect all of the research that has been going on for many years. For the average noncystic acne condition, Dr. Kohn advises his patients first and foremost to keep their hands off of their faces. Any traumatizing of the lesions can make the condition worse. So that means no picking, poking, squeezing, or fooling around with your face. So, if you're crying, use tissues, not hands to sop up the tears. And it also means that you should stay away from harsh soaps, detergents, or scrubs.

AT-HOME SOLUTIONS

But you must keep your skin clean. Dr. Kohn recommends washing two times a day with a product such as Neutrogena Acne Cleansing Soap, and then following up with an application of two-and-a-half percent, five percent, or ten percent solution of benzoyl peroxide. It is, of course, best to let your doctor decide which one you should be using even though it can be purchased over the counter. Benzoyl peroxide is a colorless lotion that is applied to the skin and can be used under makeup. Its primary function is to dry and peel the skin, which in turn clears up the existing acne. Benzoyl peroxide is very helpful as a preventative to future breakouts, and can help keep your skin quite clear in the future . . . if it is used religiously. It *really* does work; I'm never without it. You can find Benzoyl Peroxide under names such as Benoxyl 5, Benoxyl 10, Oxy 5, and Oxy 10. Just ask the pharmacist for it.

DOCTOR'S ORDERS

The other treatments that are widely accepted among dermatologists are antibiotics, which can be either applied topically or taken orally. These by-prescription-only medications include tetracycline, erythromycin, and clindamycin. Clindamycin is only available in topical form for the treatment of acne, but the other medications are available both ways.

But, as well as they work, they are not the long-awaited cure-all. And they do have side effects, which you must thoroughly discuss with your doctor beforehand. For example, tetracycline can make your skin extremely sensitive to sunlight and can even promote or encourage vaginitis.

The other prescription products that you should discuss with your doctor include Acne Topical Solution (ATS) and Retinoic Acid (Retin-A). These are topical medications, which work extremely well. ATS, a two-percent erythromycin solution, doesn't dry out your skin, really clears up existing acne, and according to Dr. Mally will actually prevent up to fifty percent of future eruptions. It is also a clear liquid, which can be applied under makeup . . . or even on a bare face. Retin-A, on the other hand, is very potent stuff and works by unplugging the blocked follicles, but you must be prepared for the generally reddened condition of your face . . . at least while you are using it.

SURE CURE?

What's all this talk we've been hearing lately about a cure for acne? Does it exist, and if so, why isn't it in wide use already?

Well, this newest media star is called 13-cis-retinoic acid, generically named isotretinoin. It is marketed by Hoffmann-LaRoche under the brand name Accutane. And yes, it does, on first glance, seem to be the long-awaited cure. It appears that this drug works directly on the sebaceous glands and the latest studies even indicate that long after the drug has been discontinued, patients remain acne free.

So, what can be bad? Well, for starters, the drug is so powerful that it should be recommended only to those suffering from the most severely recalcitrant form of cystic acne . . . acne that has been unresponsive to all other treatments, according to Dr. Kohn. Why? Because it can cause any or all of the following reactions: all-over body skin peeling, nose and mouth fissures, and even a condition known as ectropian—a downturning of the lower eyelids.

The drug should also be avoided by all women who are planning to conceive—as a safeguard against any possible fetal damage. Physicians will be warning women that this drug should only be taken in conjunction with a strictly adhered-to program of birth control.

So, while this might be a wonderful cure-all, it's a

cure-all with a catch. Dr. Kohn believes that at present it should only be prescribed for those truly suffering with a disfiguring form of acne. Period.

What does it all amount to? It *can* amount to clear skin—maybe for the first time in your life. With all of the research, new products, and treatments available these days, we no longer have to show the outward signs of acne. Just think—no more humiliating "flesh-toned" acne cream that only matched the flesh tone of the cast of *Night of the Living Dead*. So, if you've developed acne, don't sit around with it . . . kick it out the door, and get on to more important things.

TOO SENSITIVE FOR YOUR OWN GOOD

If you have sensitive skin, I'm sure it's not in great shape right now. You've been unhappy and it shows! Well, he has no right to get you into this shape, so let's fix it and show the world just how gorgeous your skin *really* is. A woman with sensitive skin may have a peaches-and-cream complexion (fair, rosy) when all is going well, which turns into a rashy mess when the least little thing happens. If that sounds familiar, you must contend with knowing that anything from a small emotional upset to using a cosmetic that is wrong for your skin type can result in another trauma: awful-looking skin.

If that sounds like you, and you have recently had a traumatic experience, chances are good that your skin is showing the results of all of this tension. You may have found that, especially now, your skin is more vulnerable than ever.

Why? Because people with sensitive skin have a

thinner, more fragile outer (keratin) layer than others. Therefore, it is less protected and will be more affected by sun, wind, soaps, detergents, temperature extremes ... in a word, anything that stimulates it. While you can't change your sensitive skin, you can take charge of it ... and yourself ... by protecting it. That means that you must treat it gently. Here's how:

- Use the mildest nondetergent soap you can find. Neutrogena and specially formulated baby soaps are great.
- Wear a sunscreen everytime you go outdoors, even if it's just to go shopping. (That keratin layer of yours is extra thin, and needs extra protection.)
- Use a moisturizer every day to protect your skin from drying, cracking, and flaking. But make sure that it is hypoallergenic ... and water based. Oil-based moisturizers can cause you to break out in acne flare-ups, if you are so prone.
- Choose hypoallergenic cosmetics and apply them sparingly, with clean cosmetic sponges. Fingers and unclean applicators contain bacteria that can undo all of the good that hypoallergenic does.
- Refrain from leaning your hand and/or the telephone receiver against your chin.
- Don't ever pick or poke at your face. Sensitive skin is more easily marked, pocked, and scarred than nonsensitive skin.

When you give yourself a facial, make it a gentle one. And that means avoid steam, vigorous massage, electric currents, and even deep vacuum-type cleaning.

PLAYING WITH THE COMBO

But what if you've got combination skin . . . it's dry as a bone in some places, spouting a gusher of oil in others, and just fine in others?

Then you've got to treat it with a combination of methods. Keep it clean with a soap such as Neutrogena® and then apply the same techniques around your face as you would if it were all the same. For example, where it's dry, apply moisturizer, where it's oily, use an astringent, where it's broken out, apply benzoyl peroxide. But no matter what shape the skin you're in is in, or what type it is, spritz it frequently with water. Remember, water is as good for your skin as love is for your head, your heart, and your hopes. And when you deprive yourself of either, you shrivel up!

12 · Eye-Do's for When He Didn't— How to Cry without Wrecking Your Eyes

Crying makes your eyes look awful. You know that. But you just can't help it, you say? It's sort of like eating one more donut, or climbing Mount Everest . . . you do it because it's there.

Well, let me tell you that I think crying is good for you—for a couple of weeks. But there are rules. First of all, don't cry alone. I mean, what's the future in it if you don't have your best friend or your mother there to hand you tissues? And anyway, crying alone—at least after the first bout—is boring and very upsetting. When you cry with a friend, at least you get a shoulder to go with your swollen eyes.

But these are the tears that you've got to get out of the way. Crying is healthy. It's a catharsis, a way to wash away all of the bad stuff that's still clogging up your

brain. So I'm going to allow you to do it for a few weeks
. . . and then no more!!! Remember, I've been through
all of this, and all I can tell you is that it *does* get better.
Really it does.

But in the meantime, you've got some crying to do,
and you may even run out of friends before you run out
of tears. So either learn to control the flow—or learn to
cry properly without wrecking your eyes.

Eye exercises can help prevent damage, and eye
packs can help turn your swollen reds into bright whites.
Here are some ways to do just that.

EYECERCISES

WIDE-EYED

To disperse accumulated liquids and reduce eye puffiness, look straight ahead into a mirror. Open your eyes
as wide as possible, without actually wrinkling your forehead. Now, relax them as much as possible in the open
position. Slowly bring the lower lids up to meet the
upper lids. Hold this position for a count of ten and then
relax. Repeat six times. Now, close your eyes and relax
completely. Let the tension drain from your entire face.
Just relax. Don't move your upper lids or squinch your
eyes. The only part of your face that will move is the
lower lid.

PRESS TO REFRESH

Many experts recommend the following exercise to reduce eye puffiness quickly. Press your index fingers
against the bridge of your nose (near the corners of the

eyes) and hold for seven seconds. Then move the fingers to just *below* the inner eye corner. Hold and press. Continue to move along pressing and holding the fingers under each section of the under eye socket. Hold and press in each spot for a count of seven. Keep moving and pressing all the way out to the temples and into the hairline. This technique really works by breaking up the edema (water retention) in the area.

M. J. SAFFON'S EYELID SAVER
Upper Lids

To save your upper eyelids from total destruction, my friend M. J. Saffon, author of numerous books, including *The Fifteen Minute A Day Natural Facelift,* has devised this eye exercise. It actually prevents sagging upper lids and, when done religiously, can restore the firmness if your lids have already begun to droop.

Cream the entire eyelid and brow bone area with a good, heavy moisturizer. Then place the four fingers of each hand over your eyelids. Press firmly at the spot where you can feel the bone. Now, raise your eyebrows sharply with the fingers while attempting to close your eyes. Try also to draw the outer corners of the eyes up while you are attempting to close your eyes. The pressure of trying to close your raised lids should feel the way you feel when you've been squinting a long time. Hold for a count of six. Relax, drop hands, and repeat the entire procedure six times.

Eye Packs for Eye Bags

Now we already know that you've spent a lot of time crying and/or not sleeping. So chances are really good that some days will find you with red, puffy, swollen eyes. You can unpuff 'em in a flash with special, easy little eye packs. Here are some favorites:

TEA FOR TEARS
(Eye Depuffer)

6 teabags

Soak six teabags in water that is still boiling hot, but which has been removed from the heat. Let the brewed tea *cool* to room temperature. Then apply three bags to each closed eye. Or you can chill the mixture in the fridge and apply them cold. If your eyes are still puffy, soak your face, eyes open, in a bowl of cold distilled water for a minute. Yes, you can come up for air when you need to.

The other products that work to unpuff eyes are potatoes, cucumbers, and ice bags. If you want to get done quickly, just apply slices of chilled veggies to your eyes, and lie down with your feet up.

BAGS FOR BAGS

If you want to get fancy you can grind up raw potatoes and tie the pieces up in a little square of cheesecloth and secure with a ribbon. Place one on each eye and lie down. Place a pillow under your feet and rest for as long as you like.

REFRESH, RELAX, DE-RED YOUR EYES

cotton balls
witch hazel

Soak cotton balls (natural cotton, not plastic cotton, please) in chilled witch hazel. Apply them to your closed eyelids. Prop your feet up with a few pillows and relax for twenty minutes.

MINT GLINT

2 fresh mint leaves
commercial eye drops

To get the sparkle back into tired, haggard-looking eyes, place a few drops of Visine® or Murine® into each eye. Then lie back and relax for a few minutes. When your eyes feel soothed somewhat, place a fresh mint leaf under each eye. Close your eyes and relax for as long as you can.

MILK BATH FOR EYES

When your eyes are really tired and swollen, apply compresses (cucumbers, cotton balls, etc.) soaked in cold milk for instant relief.

OR

Soak the cucumbers in *raw* milk (that's the kind you get at the health food store) and apply the cukes to your eyes. It actually seems to work better than pasturized milk!

ICE IS NICE

12 camomile tea bags

Take a dozen camomile tea bags and steep them in cold water. Refrigerate. Whenever you wake up to eyes that won't open, apply a chilled bag to your eyes and lie down with a pillow or, better, two pillows under your head.

Now, if you must, go and have yourself a good cry! You can feel confident that at least you can undo the damage!

Another word about crying—Unless you let yourself get into all of the unhappiness that you are feeling, you won't emerge in a few weeks or months, a happier, more vibrant lady. You must, of course, feel the pain before you can feel the anger. And then the anger, too, will go. And it will be replaced by a smarter, savvier ego to go along with your new look.

FOCUS-POCUS? NO! MEDITATING FOR WHAT YOU WANT

In this section, I've given you lots of ways to relax and de-red swollen eyes. Now here's something more off-beat, but equally useful.

While you are relaxing each day with one of the eye packs, I want you to teach yourself to use this time to focus in on what it is that you really want. Fantasize about what your next love affair will be like. Get specific. Concentrate on what your new lover will be like, how you'll feel, how happy you'll be. This sort of meditation is called focusing or visioning. It's a method of meditation, if you will, that will allow you to see what it is that you really want.

Meditate and focus on the same picture for the same amount of time each day. Believe it and within a short period of time, you will find that you have placed yourself in the right situations and the right places for making your fantasy become a reality. But you must believe it for it to really be. You cannot let any negative thoughts interfere in your meditation time. It works.

And remember, it is time now to stop focusing on what *was*. That is negative energy and will do nothing whatever to help you. So stop it. It's time.

13 · Facials without Fuss

Everybody loves a facial. But with the cost of professional facials these days, most of us can't even afford the first five minutes. So, if you'd love to luxuriate in the wonders of a facial, do it at home while you're still feeling bad. Here's how:

1. *Clean it out.*
   - Wash your hands with soap and water.
   - Apply your favorite cleanser to your face and throat with a cotton ball.
   - Using a fresh cotton ball soaked in toner, finish cleaning and refreshing the skin.

2. *Massage it in.*
   - Put a generous amount of thick face cream in the palms of your hands and massage your face

and neck (using palms only) in circular motions. .

• Pat cream gently around the eyes, never using harsh or pulling motions. Make sure cream does not get into the eyes themselves.

• Use the middle and index fingers to massage your nose and lips and all of your fingertips for the chin.

• Massage cream in with both hands for the neck. Use up-and-down motions.

3. *Steam it.*

• Steep a pot of boiling herb tea (see "Tea Totaling" for which teas work on which skin types). Place a towel over your head and around the open pot. (After it's been removed from the heat source, of course!) The towel should now resemble a tent. Remain this way until the tea is no longer steaming. (This step opens pores for the final nourishing mask.)

4. *Nourish it.*

• Apply a nourishing mask, and leave it on for about twenty minutes. Remove with lukewarm water and follow up with a good moisturizer (if your face is dry).

TEA TOTALING

To get even more from your facial, brew the special tea known to help your skin type:

Camomile: Dry and/or sensitive skin
Peppermint tea: Oily skin
Comfry root tea: Acne and broken-out skin
OR

Make your own herb tea: Add thin strips of lemon peel and rind to a pot of steeping tea. Add a teaspoon or so of marjoram and crushed mint.

FEED YOUR FACE

Now that you know how to give yourself a facial, here are a bunch of marvelous masks you can whip up from ingredients you'll probably find in the fridge, the cupboard, or the medicine cabinet. See, I told you that you wouldn't be forced to go out . . . yet! (Except to visit the hairdresser of your choice—often and well.)

Dry Skin Masks

MOISTURE MASK

½ ripe avocado
¼ cup yogurt

Peel and mash the pulp from half a very ripe avocado. Mix it till smooth with the yogurt. Apply the mixture to your face and leave it on for about fifteen minutes. Remove by rinsing with warm water.

Bonus tip—To prevent an avocado from discoloring, rinse the peeled avocado in lemon juice or a mixture of lemon juice and cool water.

ALL ALONE AVOCADO MASK

Just mash up half an avocado, and apply the pulp to your face. Leave on about fifteen minutes and remove with lukewarm water.

Oily Skin Masks

BOAST ABOUT OATS MASK

3 tablespoons oatmeal
1 tablespoon dry milk
1 egg white

Grind the oatmeal in your blender until powdery. Add the dry milk and blend some more. Mix in the egg white and apply the mixture to your face. After the mask sets (about fifteen minutes), rinse your face with soap and warm water.

Bonus tip—Mix up enough dry ingredients for several masks and store them in airtight jars or Seal-A-Meal bags. Then just add one egg white to each four tablespoons of dry premixed ingredients whenever the urge to sow your oats hits.

RAISE A FUSS YEAST MASK

Mix enough yeast with water to form a paste. Mix well and apply to your face. Leave it on twenty minutes, and then rinse with warm water.

MERINGUE MASK

1 egg, separated
juice of one lemon

Beat the egg whites till peaks are formed. Then blend it together with the strained juice of one lemon. Apply the mixture evenly to your freshly washed face, avoiding the delicate under-eye area. When the application is nearly dry, add another coating, and then another.

(The oilier your skin, the more coatings you should apply.) Now, the hard part . . . literally! Leave the hardened mask on your face for about thirty minutes without talking or moving facial muscles. Then remove it with cool water.

Bonus tip—Use the mask also to help lighten a fading tan. Or, plant the lemon seeds and grow your own facial at home!

EGG ON YOUR FACE MASK

1 egg, separated

Separate an egg. Apply the beaten yolk to your face. Let it dry and rinse well with cool water to remove. Next whip up the egg white and apply *it* to your face. When the white dries, remove by rinsing well with water.

This facial gives you a double bonus. The yolk is a good skin nourisher and the whites tighten up the skin, giving you a younger look.

SOW YOUR OATS MASK

½ cup oatmeal
1 tablespoon unprocessed honey
1 tablespoon cider vinegar
¼ cup warm water (try distilled, or spring water)

Mix it up and apply it evenly to your face and throat. Hide for ten minutes and then remove with lukewarm water. Follow up with a light moisturizer.

YOGURT (YES, YOGURT AGAIN) FACE MASK

Equal parts yogurt and honey

Simply mix it up and relax as much as possible for ten minutes. Rinse off with warm water. Eat whatever you didn't use. It's not nice to throw food away.

MAGIC LOTIONS AND POTIONS

Here they are at last . . . magic lotions and potions! No, they won't necessarily draw strange and wonderful men to your side instantly. Nor will they cause Mr. Once-Was to leave his current lady-in-waiting forever and rush to you (unless, of course, you force-feed them to a voodoo-doll likeness of his royal personage).

Well, what good *are* these lotions and potions, then? They will give you good-looking skin, for one thing, and they're cheap for another. Need more? They will give you an excuse to be so busy with your home crafts that you can't go out. So there!

Magic Cleansing Lotions

GET CUTE WITH CUKES FOR NORMAL SKIN

½ cup strained cucumbers (schmoosh in a blender first)
¼ cup milk

Mix it up and apply it to your face with cotton balls. Leave it on.

"E"-Z CLEANSER FOR DRY SKIN

Plain yogurt, scooped into your hand and spread on your face, is a terrific skin cleanser. If you have dry skin, it adds a new dimension if you puncture a vitamin E capsule and mix it into the yogurt. Remove by wiping or rinsing it off. Then splash on lots of cool water.

MILLION-DOLLAR BABY FACE ASTRINGENT
For Oily Skin

2 ounces of witch hazel
a few drops of lemon juice

Here's how to whip up this super, quick, easy (and cheap) astringent. Simply mix the ingredients together. Then refrigerate the mixture in a sterilized glass jar and use whenever the oil backs up. If you've not used an astringent before, simply moisten a cotton ball with the lotion and spread it up and around your face to sop up excess oil and grime.

ALMOND JOY SCRUB FOR ACNE/OILY SKIN

2 tablespoons ground almonds
½ teaspoon whole milk
½ teaspoon white flour

Grind up the almonds in a blender or food processor. Then mix about two tablespoons of the almond pulp with the milk and flour. Mix it around till the mixture forms a crunchy consistency. Apply to your face using a gentle circular motion. Simply rinse off with ten or more handfuls of warm water.

SLOUGH THE ROUGH SCRUB
All Skin Types, Sloughs off Dead Skin

*3 tablespoons skinned almonds (Skinned almonds? Yes,
skinned almonds!)*
1 tablespoon yogurt

Place the almonds in your blender. Blend at high speed
until they have taken a powder. Mix it up with the yogurt
and apply to your face in gentle upward strokes. Splash
with cold water to remove.

You can mix up a whole batch of powdered almonds
and store in the fridge. Then just add the yogurt whenever you've the urge to slough the roughs.

VODKA TONIC
(from Lia Schorr)

2 tablespoons honey
1 teaspoon lemon juice
4 teaspoons rosewater
5 teaspoons vodka

Mix the whole thing together and let it stand in a sterilized jar for a full week. Then use as a cleanser by applying with a cotton ball. No need to rinse.

No Frills Potions

MILK-IT CLEANSER

Just use plain milk as a cleanser—instead of soap and
water—whenever your face feels dry and irritated. Rinse
if off with mineral water, distilled water, or rosewater.

CORNMEAL CLEANSER

Just put a teaspoon or so into the palm of your hand and add enough water to form a paste. Rinse with cool water. Goodbye gunk.

PINEAPPLE APPEAL

Apply fresh pineapple slices to your face to refresh tired-looking skin. Leave on for ten minutes, splash on cool water.

AU PEAR GIRL

Or apply slices of fresh pear to your face and follow the above procedure.

14 · A Ton of Makeup Tricks to Try When You Have Enough Energy

MAKEUP TO MAKE OUT

Makeup is a glorious thing. It can disguise the myriad mistakes that nature always makes (unless you are Brooke Shields) while giving you a lift that you can always use. The best part about makeup? It lets you be a little kid again. You can hide out in your room and play with all of those wonderful pencils and crayons (unless you are Brooke Shields in which case you already *are* a kid) plus you get to erase all of your mistakes! Here, then, a bunch of wonderful tips and tricks to try while feeling sorry for yourself. You'll be so happy with all of this new experimenting that you'll even want to start going out and showing off! It's getting close to that time, anyway, you know.

Looking Better Than You Feel

If you haven't been getting much sleep lately, it's going to show. First, read "Sleep . . . Sweet Sleep" (page 45) and keep all of those tips in mind. But, if you need to look good right this second, here's a quick makeup routine that can disguise the fact that you feel rotten right this second. Remember, when you look great, you feel . . . at least a little better.

First, depuff your eyes with any of the cold compresses you just learned about. Then lie down with your feet propped up for a few minutes. (The longer the better.) Then when you are done, lie on your bed and dangle your head and arms toward the floor. (This will help to rev you up and wake you up.)

WHAT YOU'LL NEED

Powder brush
Liquid foundation
Under eye concealer
Makeup sponges
Black eyeliner pencil
Powder or gel blusher
Baby powder
Mascara
Eyelash curler
Smoky powder shadow
Lip pencil
Lipstick

THE TEN-MINUTE MAKEOVER

1. Start with a firm foundation. Most makeup artists will tell you that foundation is the most important part of any makeup routine. So, let's start at the beginning with the right foundation in the right shade.

First, choose the foundation that is right for your particular skin type. You can find moisturizing foundations, foundations with sunscreen, and foundations blended specifically for oily and normal complexion types. But, after you've found the right product, you've got to find the right shade. To do so, apply a dot to your neck, blend it in well. Does it show? Then it's not the right one for you. When you find the right shade, it will be a perfect match, you will see no line of demarcation between the foundation and your skin.

To apply your foundation like a pro, begin by applying three dots to each cheek and three to your forehead with the tip of a makeup brush handle. Then apply two dots to your nose and one on your chin. Blend well with a little makeup sponge all over your face and right into your hairline. But stay away from your neck unless you're looking for ring around the collar. (Remember, necks are for checking color only.) Finish up with a drop of foundation on your eyelids to help shadow adhere, and a drop on your lips to keep your lipstick from running on at the mouth. Blend well.

Bonus tip—Finish by washing out your sponge to keep bacteria and gunk from collecting. What does a makeup sponge do? Your sponge helps the foundation to blend smoothly and requires only half as much makeup as you'd use if you used your fingers. It also helps keep the foundation from seeping into your pores. I don't know why . . . it just does. Trust me.

2. *The rings of slattern.* I imagine by now you've got dark circles under your eyes . . . lack of sleep and stress no doubt? If foundation alone doesn't do the job, use an under-eye concealer to disguise your own personal rings of slattern. Pick a shade that is only one to two shades lighter than your normal skin tone. If your under-eye concealer is too light, you can end up looking like an albino raccoon. And you certainly don't want to trade black rings for white ones.

Apply the cream to your fingertips, then pat on around your under-eye area. Follow up with foundation.

3. *Add some color.* To find the most natural shade of blusher, pinch your cheeks. Your blusher should match that shade as closely as possible. Begin applying blusher on the highpoints of your cheekbones. Start just under the center of your eye, stroking along the cheek toward the ear. Apply in several thin coats rather than in a single heavy one. But be generous. You can stand a little color.

4. *Baby yourself.* To set your makeup, pour a tiny bit of baby talcum powder into your hand, and dip a big powder brush into it. Flick or blow away excess powder. Then softly stroke the brush over your makeup to give it a real pro finish.

5. *Play up your eyes.* Now comes the best part . . . your eyes! Use a soft eyepencil to draw a thin line from the middle of your upper lid to the outside corner.

Repeat this process below the lower lashes, smudging both lines with a cotton swab. Next, curl your lashes with an eyelash curler and apply your mascara. Apply one coat to both sides of the upper and lower lashes. Move on to the next eye and apply the same number of coats. Go back again to eye number one and repeat the process, and then repeat on the second eye. Your eyelashes will look thick, lush, and gorgeous. Finally, apply a smoky powder shadow in the crease of the lid and blend well. You will look wide-eyed, not made up.

6. *Line your lips.* Next comes the mouth. Outline your mouth with a lip pencil that matches your lipstick exactly or as closely as possible. If your lips are too thin, line just outside the natural lip line. If they are too thick, line just inside the natural lip line. Then draw an inverted V in the center of your upper lip and a regular V on the bottom lip. Draw several vertical lines around both top and bottom lips. Finally, fill in with your matching lipstick. The lines will not show at all. Blot up, reapply, and blot lightly. Your lipstick will stay stuck for hours.

7. *Set it and forget it.* If you'd like, you can further "set" your makeup by spritzing your face with mineral or distilled water. Believe it or not, that whole routine shouldn't have taken you more than ten minutes. So, you've no excuse to stay home today. You look wonderful.

EVEN QUICKER!

Ready, Set, and Glowing in Five Minutes Flat

If you're running late, because you've spent lots of time moaning . . . here's how to make up and get moving, in five minutes flat. First give your skin a tingling fresh start by gently wiping it with a cleanser-soaked, purse-sized tissue. Follow with a moisturizing rose or bronze-tinted face gel just for the sheer blush of it. It will give you just the hint of healthy color you need. Then apply a tinted lip gloss. Finish up by lining, shadowing, and contouring your eyes with one eye pencil that does it all . . . or . . . if you prefer, dab on cream shadow with its own sponge applicator. For a final flourish, brush your lashes with a waterproof mascara, and your hair with a natural bristle brush. While this isn't a complete makeover, it is an alternative to facing the world naked . . . faced. So, ready, set . . . Glow!

MAKE UP LIKE A PRO: TIPS, TRICKS, AND EMERGENCY REPAIRS

Eye-lusions

Are you aware that most people don't have perfectly spaced eyes? It's true. The experts say that the ideal width is one eye width between your eyes. To find out whether your eyes are too closely spaced or too wide apart, try this: Place a ruler horizontally on the bridge of your nose. Line up the front edge of the ruler with the outer corner of one eye. Measure the width of that eye, from the outer corner to the inner corner. Mark the measurement on the ruler.

Now, with the ruler on the bridge of your nose, line up the edge of the ruler with the inner corner of the eye you just measured. If your eye-width measurement marked on the ruler extends beyond the inner corner of your other eye, your eyes are spaced too closely together. If the measurement falls short, they're too far apart. Now that you know, here's how to create the illusion of perfection . . . .

CLOSE SET

If your eyes are closely set and you'd like to look a bit more wide-eyed, you'll need three shades of the same hue of eye shadow. (light, medium and dark). Smooth the medium shade over your lids. Stroke the light shade under your brows and place the darkest shade from the middle of you eyelids towards the outer edges. Blend well. Voilà!

SPACED OUT

But what about eyes that are too widely spaced? Again, you'll need three shades of the same hue of eye shadow. In this case, the medium shade goes over your lids, the lightest shade under your brows, but here's the difference—the darkest shade is placed in the inner corners bringing your eyes closer together. Blend all of the edges of the shadows well.

LASH DASH

Lashes too light? Well, you can always use mascara, and I do mean always. Or you can have your lashes dyed. It saves lots of time. But get it done *professionally!* Now or as soon as you're ready.

BIGGER AND BETTER

Want your eyes to appear bigger than they really are? Try this professional model's trick: Apply a pale color shadow from the lashes to the brow. Smudge a brown-toned shadow onto the crease line for contouring. Finish up by curling lashes with an eyelash curler and then applying mascara.

MORE CLOSE CALLS

Another trick that models use to make their eyes appear to be spaced further apart: Blend a tiny dot of white eye shadow between the inner corner of your eye and the bridge of the nose. Then apply your colored shadow from the center of your top eyelids outward.

PROMINENT LIDS . . . PERMANENT SOLUTION

If you've prominent lids, lucky you! But some people don't like them. So if you've got 'em and don't want 'em, remember this rule: Light emphasizes and dark takes away. So, if you've prominent lids, keep away from light shadows, or you'll end up with eyes that look like the headlights of a '57 Cadillac. Stick with brown-toned shadows and apply them from the lash line to the crease line. If you'd love a little color, too, just use a little on the outer corners.

WHAT'S MY LINER

Heavy eyeliner dates you, and makes you look older than you are. Here's the newest way to line your eyes: Just dot it on all along the base of your lashes and then smudge it with a cotton swab. The look? Smokey instead of burned out!

TOO DEEP FOR YOUR OWN GOOD

Do you think that your eyes are too deep set? Bring them out with a light pastel shadow on the lids. Wear lots of mascara and concentrate your efforts on the lashes in the center.

RUNNING IN THE WRONG CIRCLES

If you've got circles under your eyes, you can try this: Use a neutralizer to even out uneven skin tone. Use a lavender-based toner if you've got sallow skin and a green neutralizer if you have ruddy or florid skin. Dot it on lightly with the tail end of a makeup brush under your eyes, and around laugh lines . . . wherever you need to correct color. Blend gently . . . up and out. Apply foundation over the neutralizer and no one will know you've been, well, you know.

BROW WOW

As you know, your eyebrows can give expression to your whole face. We've all seen the ladies who have overpowering brows, or pencil-thin brows, frowning brows, and brows that are drawn on so high that they look perpetually in shock. Well, the truth is, that you probably look best with your own brow shape. So, why not let them grow in? It will take you about three months. While they are growing in, use facial bleach on the new hairs to keep you from looking as though your eyes are growing a beard. After they've grown in all the way, pluck out only the real scraggly hairs. From *under* brows only. Then train your brows to do what you want them to by rubbing a clean toothbrush over a bar of moist soap. Brush your brows in the direction you want them to take.

For brows that are too light, use a brow brush or clean toothbrush. Rub the brush over a cake of powder eye shadow (in hair color, please . . . not blue) and brush a bit of color onto your brows. Or you can have your brows dyed in the salon.

For brows that are too dark, dip your brush into some loose face powder and lightly apply to brows. Or you can have them lightened up at the salon if you have your hair colored.

TWEEZER EASER

To take the pain out of plucking, try this: Smooth a bit of Vaseline® petroleum jelly over the area to be tweezed, and place a moist, hot towel over that. Press gently to open the pores and tweeze with ease.

INSIDE TRACK

Here's a quickie that really has impact. To make your eyes and your eyelashes look lush and gorgeous, rim the *inside* of the upper lashline under the lashes with an eyeliner pencil. It's like track lighting for your lashes!

MASCARA POWER

To thicken your eyelashes and make mascara stick, dust your lashes with baby powder or face powder before you put your mascara on.

TIGHT-LIPPED LOOK

If your lips are too thick, apply your foundation onto your lips. Then use your pencil to rim just inside the natural lipline. Neutral colors work better with this trick than bright colors.

DOT TO DOT

Here's another way to create a gorgeous mouth: Place a dot at the top of each peak of each lip, with a lip pencil. Place identical dots parallel to them on the bottom lip. Then simply draw your lipline from the corners of the mouth to the dots.

NOSE GAYS

Have you ever asked yourself: Why has this nose chosen to take up residence on my face? Well, if you aren't contemplating cosmetic surgery, you should be contemplating cosmetic camouflage. But, first, realize that one of the best ways to camouflage a flaw is to play up an asset. For example, if you hate your nose, play up your eyes. But that doesn't mean that you can't camouflage a bad nose with other makeup tricks. Here's how:

To minimize a long nose, apply shading two or three tones darker than your skin . . . to the tip and base of your nose. Then blend. Your nose too broad? Use the shader along the sides of your nose and blend. Then, using a white highlighter, draw a thin line from the top of your nose . . . (just in the center between your brows) . . . straight down to the tip. Blend again. You can even diminish a hooked nose by using darker shader on the bump itself, and applying the highlighter just underneath it. For a crooked nose, shade the side of your nose that is turned *toward* your cheek. Next, using the highlighter, draw a thin, straight line down the center of your nose, *but* do *not* follow the curve. Now, whoever said . . . a nose, is a nose . . . is *the* nose you have to be stuck with?

CHEEKY

Them Bones

Have you ever looked in the mirror at them bones, them bones, them cheekbones and wished they'd grow . . . just a little? Well, very few people were born with great cheekbones. So, if you aren't Katherine Hepburn (or Audrey Hepburn), and don't have wonderful prominent cheekbones, don't despair. While you may never grow great bones, you can fake great bones with a little makeup magic. Here's how:

First, find out where they are! To do this, place your fingertips onto the tops of your cheekbones and feel for structure and placement. To make your cheekbones appear more prominent, try applying a light highlighting cream just above them. Blend well. Then place your blush just below the cheekbones and extend it out toward the temple. What you've done is create an illusion by making the cheeks appear to recede and the cheekbones appear to protrude.

Another model's trick is to place blush above the cheekbones and a brownish contouring powder in what should be the hollows of the cheeks. If you don't have hollows, contouring powder will make it look as though you do!

• Want a healthy sunny look without the sun? Brush blusher onto your face where it would get touched by the sun . . . the nose, the cheeks, the tip of your chin.

SPLIT-SECOND BEAUTY

Okay, fine. You make it out of the house looking great in the morning, but by midday you look beat up again. Here then . . . some quick revver uppers for the midday droops: That's the time when your eyes get wet and you *really* want to call him. Don't. Go get gorgeous instead.

To freshen your face during the day, splash it with warm water, then spritz it with cold mineral water. If you work, you might try keeping a can or even a plant mister in the office refrigerator for this purpose. For a quick makeup redo, simply add a dab of lip gloss to the bottom lip and a sweep of blusher from the highest point of the cheekbone outward toward the temple. You'll be amazed at how much more vibrant and lively you'll look in an instant!

If you find that your skin begins to feel grimy around midday, give it—and you—a mini cleansing with a damp cotton ball, wiping oil and grime from cheeks, forehead, and nose. Follow with a light dab of moisturizer for dry skin or a blotting lotion for oily. Redo foundation and blush. Add more lip color, and you'll feel terrific!

TWO-FACED MAKEUP

Are you twofaced? If not, you should be. At least as far as your makeup is concerned. In fact, every woman should learn to make up her face in *two* separate ways, one for evening and one for school or work.

Your Work Face

The first rule to keep in mind is that fluorescent lighting, which is the mainstay of offices and schools . . . emphasizes everything that is wrong with your skin and makeup. A face that may look perfectly made up in the gentle light of your home may look garishly overdone or childishly underdone at work.

For example, if your skin tends to be normally sallow, use a foundation with pink tones, which will help to tone down the greenish hues and build up the rosy ones. If your skin is ruddy, on the other hand, apply a green-tinted moisturizer to your face and neck *before* you make up. This little trick will keep you in the pink . . . not *over* it!

MAKING EYE CONTACT: SPECIAL TIPS FOR CONTACT LENS WEARERS

Maybe it's time for a change in the way the world sees you . . . and the way in which you see the world. Have you thought about trading in your glasses for contacts? Well, if you think that you've been spending too much

---

time hiding behind oversize glasses, it's time to give some serious thought to contacts. It really is one of the most dramatic ways to change the way you look without surgery. And in case you've ever thought about it—yes you can use contacts for strictly cosmetic purposes. You *can* change your eye color from dark to light or vice versa. Boy, that would shake up you-know-who when he runs into you!

Cosmetic lenses, according to Dr. Harry Hollander of New York's Sight Improvement Center, are fitted in the same way that regular lenses are fitted, but differ in a few ways. For example, the fit is tighter so that the lens fits snugly to keep the iris covered. Therefore, wearing time is more limited.

The lens "pupil," however, is colorless, which allows for clear vision. But since it doesn't adjust to light the way your own pupil does, there can be slight vision impairment at times.

As of this writing, "colored" contacts are available only in hard lenses, and do cost more than other correcting lenses.

It's worth thinking about, but maybe it's part of the fantasy.

Making Up for Contacts

If you are a contact-lens wearer, and have had trouble with smeared makeup because of eye watering, keep these tips in mind:

- Look for fragrance-free eye makeup, particularly mascara.
- If you are switching from glasses to contacts, you will need to change your eye makeup. Your eyes will

no longer be framed by glasses and, if you're wearing magnifying lenses, will no longer appear larger. Go for more dramatic makeup. Or go for a whole makeover.

• If possible, wait twenty minutes or so after waking to put your lenses in. This will allow the mild edema, or water retention, that follows a night's sleep a chance to clear.

• Insert or remove lenses at a table with your mirror lying prone, and not over a sink. This procedure not only gives you better leverage, but it cuts the chances of losing a lens down the drain.

• Never clean lenses with anything but recommended solutions. Lens plastic can absorb organic solvents (such as soaps and detergents) and could release them in your eye.

15 · Body Shapers

THE WEIGHT YOU TAKE

Fighting Off the Fattie Who May Be Lurking Inside You

Here it is again . . . the urge to splurge on several hundred Ring Dings, three cartons of Heavenly Hash, and an entire pork roast at one sitting. Let's face it, when depression strikes, hunger mounts. It's the old instant grats come to pay a call. Well, now is *not* the time to indulge yourself . . . not in *food* anyway. It's bad enough that you are feeling blue without feeling bloated.

But why does your appetite become gargantuan when you're upset? Well, that's because hunger, or more precisely, food, is one of your earliest nurturing memories. FOOD = COMFORT = CARED FOR = LOVE! So, naturally, when you are unhappy, you may tend to regress to these primal, and primary nurturing memories. And food becomes the regression vehicle. Unfortunately, what's on your mind can . . . and probably *will* . . . end up on your hips. (But food doesn't have to be eaten in great abundance to act as the regression vehicle.) You can also regress to another developmental stage and not eat at all.

Here's basically how the whole thing works, according to Dr. Stuart Berger, author of *The Southampton Diet,* and a doctor with a weight-control practice in New York. While food *is* a first source of nurturing pleasure, it later becomes one of the first sources of autonomy expression for children. You see, a child must eat what's given her at home (or face the general round of bickering, cajoling, and fighting), but when she leaves the house, Mom can no longer control what's eaten. She *can* throw her lunch away at school, she *can* eat an ice cream on the way home. Voila! Instant autonomy!

So, it's interesting to remember that at any given time during your recovery period, you may be faced with these two conflicting preprogrammed mind sets. You may want to eat to feel satisfied (nurtured) and you may want to eat to express your autonomy (from the dashing desperado?). Tough problem, yes, but not unsolvable once you recognize it.

In other words, it's the old "I'll show him "routine." It goes something like this: "I'll get so fat that he'll think that I can't take care of myself and he'll come back and do it for me." Or maybe it's the old "He can't tell me what to do anymore, therefore I will eat thirty-seven Big Macs. Nna, Nna, Nna, Nna."

While it *is* instantly gratifying, it is a short-lived form of gratification . . . one that will turn sour every time you look at your body. Now, that's not to say that every binge is a bad binge. Food is, after all, a wonderful, delightful way to pass the time. But, you've got to learn to indulge yourself differently, with other means.

One way to indulge yourself is by taking extra good care of yourself and your body. Remember, your body doesn't come in polyester, and if you continually gain and lose weight, it will show . . . in wrinkles, excess skin and stretch marks. All of which are permanent unless you have surgery. Even with stretch marks, you've got to have enough excess skin for the surgeon to remove in the first place.

So, let's begin, *not* with a strictly adhered-to diet plan, but with a whole new way of looking at the way in which you eat. Look closely, now and here's what you'll see:

MOOD FOODS/FOOD MOODS

Did you know that you are not only what you eat, but also how you feel? Food, you see, can help you not only to stay on your diet, but to stay happier and become less depressed . . . at all times. It's true. Recently, medical and nutritional experts have found that certain foods actually do affect your moods. My friend, Dr. Stuart Berger, whom I've mentioned earlier, gave the world a great big hug when he first introduced (for public consumption) his lists of happy and sad foods. Here then are some of the mood levelers (good guys) and depression raisers (bad guys) you should be on the alert for:

Bad-Mood Food (Depression and anxiety promoters)	Good-Mood Food (Mood-levelers)
Chianti wine	Turkey
Cola drinks	Unripened cheese
Aged cheese	Yogurt
Coffee	Pineapple
Chocolate	Milk
Tea	Oranges
Marbled meats	Green leafy veggies
Mayonnaise	Lean red meat
Pickled herring	Organ meats
Chick-peas	White wine (in tiny quantities)
Sugar	Strawberries
Lentils	Brown rice
Salt	Chicken
Sour cream	Eggs
Lobster	Lemons
Beer	Spinach
	Cantaloupe

And the interesting part is that if you look closely at this list you will notice another pattern emerging. The bad mood foods are also the ones (with the exception of coffee and tea, which contain caffeine) that are whopping high in calories.

A Word About Anorexia

Of course, if you have the opposite reaction, and just don't feel like eating at all, you might be concerned that you are becoming anorexic.

According to Dr. Berger, an anorexic is not an

overly enthusiastic dieter, or even someone who is temporarily too upset to eat. An anorexic follows a very clear-cut pattern.

For example, anorexics are usually fourteen-to eighteen-year-old girls who suffer from loss of appetite originating in the nervous system, which doesn't mean that the problem is *restricted* to this group.

They may also have an obsessive preoccupation with a slight or nonexistent overweight condition, and while they may not eat or may *pretend* to eat, they can nonetheless keep up a manic pace and may eventually even stop menstruating. If you suspect that you have reached such a stage or are really on your way . . . it's essential that you see a doctor immediately. Only a doctor can diagnose and treat this condition.

But here's the good news: Anorexia is the very rare exception, and it does have a very high recovery rate.

DIETING WHATNOTS

Great Expectations

Okay, you've taken a look and have really decided this time that you want to be thin. There's no getting around it. You want to look like a million and you want to feel like it again. My God, does anything make you feel better than having a body that's in great shape? And just think . . . you'll have this great body and guess whom you'll run into when he least expects it!!

In fact, wouldn't it be a good idea to get some extra exercise by walking to the stores you know he frequents? Hah! Will he be sorry.

But first let's put your ideas into perspective. Remember, slow and steady wins the race. The longer it takes to come off the longer it will stay off. Dieting crashes and crazes don't work because they only make you lose excess fluid, which comes back again. If you've extra fluids that you want to lose, eat asparagus and drink tea. Take 1000 units of vitamin E and stay away from caffeine every day to keep premenstrual edema (water retention, swollen breasts) to a minimum.

But mostly, remember you didn't become over-weight overnight and you won't become thin overnight either (it will happen, eventually). If you have great ex-pectations (which are also unrealistic expectations), you may find that once you lose a couple of pounds you just can't, won't, or plain hate the diet. So stay away from fads, and stick to a decent diet plan that is realistic and practical.

Dieting Defeatist

Or perhaps you are a dieting defeatist. You are if you try every new miracle diet on the market, announcing to the world, "This time it's for real!!" You also love all of the catch phrases like "The No-Diet Diet," and the "The Eat All You Want Diet," "The Drinker's Diet," and "The Gorger's Diet." You may, in fact, not lose any weight on these diets, but for sure you'll lose your money and pos-sibly your mind. You'll also find that while you are always on a diet, you never lose any weight.

Why? Because if you are a dieting defeatist, you always find something wrong with each diet, eventually. "It's too complicated," or "too exotic," or "too boring," or "too restrictive," or "too expensive." And for fad diets, you may be right. If they really did work, you wouldn't see a new diet book on the market every two minutes. Everyone in the world would just stick to that perfect diet.

But even if you do find the perfect diet, you may cheat. And one splurge is enough for the D-D. You lose hope, lose face, and give up. If you recognize yourself in this category, then admit it. The only diet miracle you'll ever find is the one you'll discover when you let the thin person hiding inside of you come out. And that will happen with a long-term, sensible diet plan and a long-term commitment to change your cheating ways.

DIETING TIPS AND TRICKS TO LIVE BY

Now that you know a bit about why you may want to eat your way through a Carvel store, let's nip your grab-bag reflex in the bud. Here are a bunch of ways to do just that:

- Slow down the rate at which you eat. The faster you eat, the more you'll eat and the more you'll gain. Remember, it takes twenty minutes for the brain to let the stomach know that it's full.
- Figure out how many calories you need a day to reach and then maintain a certain weight and stick with it. Here's how it works: An inactive person needs ten to twelve calories per pound of body fat to maintain that weight. An active person needs fifteen calories per pound. Therefore, a person weighing 120 pounds needs about 1200 calories if she is inactive and about 1800 calories if she is active.
- Exercise, if possible, before you eat. Exercise actually suppresses the appetite.

• If you become ravenous and must eat, don't. Set a bell timer for ten minutes. By that time your hunger may have passed. If it hasn't, eat something nutritious and small. Remember, nutritious foods actually satisfy you longer than nonnutritious foods simply by virtue of their makeup.

• Condiment rule: Those that are used by the pinch (dill, onion powder, parsley), the teaspoon (mustard), or the drop (vanilla) are better for your diet than those used by the tablespoon (ketchup, tartar sauce).

• Drink an eight-ounce glass of water before each meal. It will help to give you a feeling of fullness.

• Be prepared for emergencies. Stock up and prepare foods that give you bulk without bulge. Carrot sticks, cucumbers, and celery sticks will give you the sensation of eating. And if they are prepared ahead of time, they will be as easy to grab as a potato chip.

• Choose foods for meals which are harder to chew and more complicated to eat, so it will take you longer to finish. For example, a lobster takes longer to get through than lasagna. You can wipe out a pound of lasagna in the amount of time it takes just to *find* the meat in a lobster claw.

• When you just can't stop thinking about food, go into your bedroom, strip down to your skin, and stand in front of a full length mirror. Then watch yourself as you attempt to eat. Chances are good that you won't be able to do it.

• When faced with lunchtime decisions, try a sprinkling of lemon juice or parmesan cheese instead of salad dressing. Choose a slice of pizza over a burger (200 calories as opposed to 400), go for grilled fish instead of fried. For dessert (if you must), have a piece of fresh fruit or some fresh berries instead of a piece of pecan pie.

• Count chews. If you normally chew twenty times, make it thirty.

• Try to be the last person finished. Always.

• Don't ever mention to your parents that you are dieting, especially when you are having a meal with them. They will immediately revert to the starving people of Europe technique. This will not only make you feel guilty . . . it will make you feel thin.

• When dining with others (and especially when eating food prepared by the host), learn to camouflage the fact that you aren't eating everything offered. Do so by taking small portions, pushing your food around with your fork, gesturing while speaking, praising the meal. Do whatever you have to do, but don't eat it all, and don't let them know that you can't or won't.

• Going to a party? Good for you! It's about time! But stick with your diet by sticking with crudités . . . and don't dunk them. Offer to bring a specialty of your own, and then make it something you can eat. Stay away from anything that looks as if it's been prepared with cheese. Cheese can be murderously high in calories and you won't even know what you're eating. Alcohol is murder, too. So stick with a white wine spritzer and then nurse just one or two all night. (When it's made in a tall glass with lots of soda and ice, it will give you lots to nurse.)

• Think of finger foods as fat foods. We all know that it would take the will power of Gandhi to eat one potato chip or one cookie. Just stay away.

• Don't keep junk in the house. If you think you must because you have kids, think again. Kids don't need junk any more than you do. They will learn in time that if there just aren't any brownies around, an apple will do just as well. Believe me, by stocking the house with junk, you are not only reverting to your mother's starving people ploy, but you are repeating it to your kids.

• Love soup? Then remember that dieters should only have soup that is clear enough to see through.

• Packaged "diet food" often contains the same number of calories as regular food. The only difference is that they use an artificial sweetener in place of sugar. It still will contain a ton of fluid-retaining sodium (and bloating helps increase depression).

• Keep a food diary and write down every morsel of food you consume. And that includes everything you even taste. Keep a regular diary, too. Go back and read it when you are happy again.

• Keep salt out of your food and on the table. Most American diets are built on pillars of salt. If your family or guests want salt, they can add it themselves. The average American consumes two to four teaspoons a day, which adds up to fifteen pounds a year!!

• Try to choose fresh foods over prepared foods. Most prepared foods contain massive amounts of sugar, which can wreck all of your intentions. For example, a tablespoon of ketchup contains a teaspoon of sugar!

• Keep in mind that only 100 extra calories a day more than your body needs will cause you to gain ten pounds a year! (That's one extra can of cola daily, or a few cookies.)

• Keep your diet to yourself. The most boring dinner conversation in the world to your nondieting friends is your diet. Your trials and tribulations are mistimed subjects to people about to have a sumptuous meal. Think about it this way: If you have a friend who is a proselytizing vegetarian, doesn't it bring you to the point of hostility when she brings the subject up as you are about to dive into a burger? Well, it's the same with nondieters. In fact, your stories may even force them to dangle a cream puff under your nose. And then good-bye good intentions! Besides, they are already listening to your love problems. Enough is enough.

• Finally, don't feel alone. I know that when you feel fat, you think that no one in the world has ever looked as awful as you feel. But, it's not true. We've all felt that way at some point in our lives. In fact, about 50 million Americans are at least ten pounds overweight. While that might not sound like a lot of weight, it *is* a lot of people! So become *obsessed,* if you must, with your new goal, which is more than just a new bathing suit . . . it's a whole new way of life. After all, we all know by now just what the best revenge is!

16 · Exercises to Do When You Can't Bear to Leave Your Bed

If you've taken to your bed (and who doesn't when misery strikes?), but feel guilty just watching your thighs grow, you can exercise without ever having to leave your cozy little bed . . . or at least without leaving your cozy bedroom. Here are some of my favorite ways to do just that:

STRETCH THAT SPINE

Begin to feel better and more energized by stretching that spine! While you're still in bed, bring your arms straight back over your head. Part your feet slightly. Stretch and elongate your spine slowly (very slowly) for about a minute or two. Ahhh, it feels divine. Then while you're still lying on your back, place your arms at your sides and slide your leg up and down . . . bending your knee . . . for a count of two. Do each leg ten times to a slow, normal tempo to start. Now, that's a real circulation revver and body mover. And *that,* my dear, is probably the best thing you can do for your body in bed . . . at least this week!

BEDTIME·BODY BUDDIES

Now, after you've done all of that stretching, try bicycling in your bed. You know, the old bicycle, don't you? If not, here's how: Lie on your back and lift your legs, supporting your back by placing your hands at the base of your spine. Now, move those legs as quickly as you can in a bicycle motion. Believe it or not, it really works!

BEDROOM BALLET

Leigh Welles, a gorgeous woman who leads exercise classes in her New York studio, has devised a whole series of exercises which she calls ballet in the bedroom. They really work and they are fun to do. And, as Leigh says, it's never too early or too late to start reshaping your body through exercise. Begin with these two exercises twice a week, at least. Oh, you'll have to get out of bed, but only as far as the bedroom door!

BARRE THE DOOR
For Hips and Thighs

Instead of a ballet barre, you'll use the doorknob for this one. Here's how: Close the door. Stand sideways to the door. Put your feet together, holding onto the door handle with one hand. Rise up on the balls of your feet, pull away from the door, raising your arm over your head and toward the door, then stretch into a crescent moon. Pull in your stomach, pull up your knees and thighs. You should feel the weight lifting out of your hips and stomach. Reverse motion and return to the starting position. Turn around and repeat on the other side. Feeling good? Then feel great . . . next time try it *au naturel!*

TUMMY TIGHTENER

To tighten your tummy and thighs, hold onto the knob of your bedroom door, standing sideways. Raise your hand as if to salute. Then stretch your fingers forward as far as you can. Reach as close to the floor as you can get. Keep the weight on the bottom of your feet, not your legs. Pull in your stomach muscles, pull your chest to your chin, and contract the stomach muscles as strongly as possible. Now you should be bent forward in a U. Reverse motions as you come up, returning to the salute position. Rise up on the balls of your feet, keeping the knees stretched and tummy tight. Move your arm to two inches behind you toward the ceiling with your eyes following your raised hand. Reverse and follow the same procedure on the other side. Do as many as you are comfortable with.

ISOMETRIC TONERS

Isometrics are wonderful exercises to do when you've taken to your bed. They not only work, but they won't cause you to feel more exhausted than when you started. While isometrics alone won't do the job on your body for your whole life, they will work for you now . . . and they will work forever in conjunction with a regular exercise program. And, with isometrics, you are the judge of your own capacity. The following exercises are designed to tone up your face and body in specific areas. What you should do is hold each contraction to the maximum intensity for a slow count of six. Be sure when you are doing each exercise that you work only on one muscle group at a time. Here's how:

BETTER BREASTS

Sit up in your bed. Then lock the fingers of both hands together, with nails of each hand pressing against the pads at the base of the fingers of the other hand. Place your hands, elbows out, against your chest, the back of your left hand against your chest, the fingers of the right hand facing out. Then attempt to pull the locked hands in opposite directions. Hold and relax. Do as many as you are comfortable with.

BREAST FIRMER

Sit up straight. Then cup one hand over the other. Place your arms out, hands resting on your chest, with the knuckles of the hand facing upward and just under the chin. Now, squeeze the hands together as tightly as you can. Rest, relax, and repeat as many times as you are comfortable with.

SUCK IN THAT GUT!

For tighter stomach muscles, get out of bed . . . just for a minute! Then stand up straight with your arms at your sides. Suck in your stomach muscles and hold as tightly as you possibly can for a slow count of six. Breathe out, relax, repeat.

FACIAL FIRMERS

• To firm up eyes, open your eyes as widely as possible. Then hold for a count of six while looking up, down, left, and right.
• To firm up cheeks and mouth, form the lips as though you were whistling. Hold tightly for a full count of six. Do this exercise vigorously.
• To firm up the neck, contract the muscles on the left side of the neck while holding the head very still. Keep pulling until you feel the chest muscles move upward. Keep your mouth closed. Hold for a full count. Relax and repeat on the other side.
• For a smoother forehead, place your balled-up fists against your forehead, with the thumbs on your forehead. Press as hard as you can for the full count of six.

STAND ON YOUR HEAD WITHOUT GETTING OUT OF YOUR BED

When you are in the middle of a personal energy crisis, do as professional models do when they feel a fast fade coming on: Stand on your head!

Yes, yes, I told you that you could stay in bed, so here goes: Lie on the bed face down, with your head and shoulders hanging over the side. Be sure to place your hands firmly on the floor for support. Stay put for a few minutes. Then get up slowly. In a short time, you should be feeling snappier and sharper! An added bonus? It gives instant relief to swollen feet. Now, that's a real two-fer.

STRESS FOR SUCCESS?

Finally, a word . . . and a tip about all of this stress that you've been going through. Did you know that you can actually draw vitality from stress? And that you can use stress creatively to make you look better and feel better?

But to use stress, instead of being used *by* it, you've got to learn to make it work for you. And then leave it behind. If you are feeling particularly stressed right this minute, lie down on your bed and imagine yourself floating down a lake on a raft, with the sun on your skin and a cool drink in your hand. Try to relax every muscle in your body. When you are ready to return to reality, count backward slowly from five to one. And finally, before we end this chapter, I can only say that if you begin to think of your obstacles as challenges, you'll be able to use the adrenalin pumping through your veins to give you a whole new competitive edge . . . not a nervous retreat.

Guess what? It's time to get out of bed, and get on with living!

EXERCISES TO DO WHEN YOU JUST DON'T WANT TO GO OUT

By now you *have* to be feeling better. You should even begin to feel *much* better. You like the new you that's slowly emerging, right? Good! Now, let's get busy with some firmers and shapers that you can do right in your own home. I know you aren't quite ready for the big move yet (to the outdoors), but it's coming . . . it's coming.

Begin by incorporating body-revving activities right into your normal everyday activities. For example, you can begin to learn how to use your body in different ways. Start out by propping your leg up on the sink and stretching it out when you brush your teeth. Or, if you've enough room direct it behind you like a ballet dancer, and keep it level. Reverse the legs and hold.

Here's another great trick: Get your metabolism moving by putting your pantyhose on while lying down on the bed. Remove them in the evening in the same way.

Legsercises

THIGH HIGHS

If you wish that your thighs would go and grow on someone else's body, take heart. Here are some sure-fire thigh slimmers. Repeat them religiously, and in a few weeks you'll have legs that just won't quit, instead of legs that just won't quit growing! Do one or several of the following every day:

• Stand with your feet facing out and your legs spread as far apart as you comfortably can. Then with your hands on your hips, squat down and begin bouncing up and down, getting as close to the floor as you can. Keep it up for one full minute. While this exercise is hard to do, just keep thinking, "Only twenty more seconds to go," and so on. After what seems like an eternity, the minute will be up.

• Sit on a chair, hands at the sides of the seat for balance, feet on the floor. Raise your left leg waist high and return. Repeat with the other leg. Do as many as you are comfortable with, increasing the amount every day. And guess what? In a few weeks, you'll be thrilled that those thighs *do* belong on your legs.

• To firm outer thighs, do leg lifts. Begin by lying on your side with your knees bent in front of you. Stretch the top leg out straight. Keeping your foot parallel to the floor, raise and lower your leg. Do this ten times on each side to start. Gradually increase the number of leg lifts each day.

• To firm loose thighs, lie down on your back on the floor. Rest your arms comfortably at your sides. Bend your knees and draw your heels up as close to your backside as you can. Then spread your knees as far out as possible, making sure to keep your feet flat on the floor. Then slowly bring your knees back together again, and spread them out, again. If you can, do this one at least twenty times.

• More tight thighs: Lie on the floor on your side, leaning up on your elbow. Now flex your foot on the side facing the ceiling, and bring it forward toward your waist. Raise your foot halfway up to your body and lower it again. Do this twenty to thirty times if you can. Now raise that same leg, flex the toe up toward the ceiling, and raise and lower the leg twenty to thirty times. Repeat the process on the other side, resting between each exercise.

WAIST CINCHERS: EXERCISES TO NIP THE WAIST

TWIST AND DON'T SHOUT

Ready to trim that waistline? Then try this: Stand with your arms raised to shoulder level (you should now look like a T) and your legs slightly apart. Then simply twist from side to side, pausing briefly at each position. For an added extra, do this exercise while holding weights.

Bonus weights tips—Want to experiment with weights without going to the expense? Use two-pound cans of veggies instead. Just hold the cans in each hand and double the benefit of any exercise that requires arm movements.

SWING AND SWAY

Stand with feet apart, holding a stick over your head. Then simply bend from side to side. Start with ten swings a day, and increase it as you can.

PULL AND PUSH

Stand straight, holding your two-pound can in one hand and holding onto the back of a kitchen chair with the other. Then lean your body outward and raise your arm. Twirl your wrist six times. Straighten yourself out and repeat. Switch to the other side and do the same thing. Do as many as you are comfortable with.

TUMMY TIGHTENERS

Have you forgotten what your feet look like? Then it's time to get your tummy into shape. And here's the good news: Your tummy is actually pretty easy to keep in shape, once you get it into shape. All you need to do is find the exercise regimen that works for you and stick with it. Here are some great ones to start with.

GET BENT

Lie flat on your back on the floor, making sure that you've a secure footing, by taking care to tuck and lock your feet under a bed, or even a dresser.

Then bend your knees and place your hands behind your head. Proceed with your bent-knee sit-ups. If you can manage twenty-five to start, it would be wonderful. If you exhale as you sit up and inhale as you return to the starting position, you'll find that your stamina is increased too.

LEG RAISERS

This is one exercise where you can actually feel your tummy tightening, even as you go. Lie flat on your back on the floor. You can ball your fists up and place them under your backside for extra support. Then inhale as you bring your legs straight up. Exhale slowly, as you lower your legs. When you've reached to about six inches off the floor, hold them there to a count of ten. Raise legs again as you inhale. Ten to start . . . increase as you can.

HOP TO IT! JUMPING ROPE: THE OVERALL BODY SHAPER

If you think that jumping rope is kidstuff, then you may be unaware that ten minutes of rope jumping does as much for your cardiovascular system as thirty minutes of jogging . . . and you don't even have to leave the house! Jumping rope also helps to firm up calves, thighs, and hips while increasing your stamina and coordination.

All you need are flat shoes and cotton socks to absorb perspiration, and a good bra to prevent tissue damage. The only other requirement? The right-size rope. To find out what's right for you, stand on the middle of the rope. The handles should reach your underarms.

To begin, stand inside the loop with your feet together. Pull the rope ends up. They should stretch to just under your arms. Keep the rope close to your body with your hands (not your arms) doing most of the work.

Jumping action should be on the balls of the feet, rather than the soles. Bend a little at the ankles, knees, and hips. Don't jump sky high . . . about an inch off the floor is best for speed. Choose a hard surface to jump on, because it will "bounce back" with you. And although you probably jumped barefoot as a kid, experts say that you should wear well-cushioned athletic shoes as an adult. And finally, take it short, take it slow, and take it easy. It's a gradual buildup to jumping five minutes a day, five times a week that you're after.

BONUS ROPE TRICKS

To help you learn the ropes before you start:

- Use the right equipment. Try a ball-bearing exercise rope for the best balance.
- Jump rope in an unobstructed area, with a ceiling height of eight to ten feet (you'll need a higher ceiling if you are very tall).
- Keep your hands close to your body and skip lightly; spring at the ankles rather than the knees.
- Skip alternately with the right and left foot for sixty seconds. Shoot for a cadence of 120 counts per minute (a count is each time either foot hits the floor). Rest for one minute and repeat.
- Try doing the above exercise with your arms held away from your body, to firm upper arms and chest muscles.

17 · Exercises to Do When You Are Ready to Go Out Again!

SHAPING UP AWAY FROM HOME

Shaping up used to be done in secret. Now the whole world shapes up in public view. And so will you. You are already getting gorgeous, and it's time you started *getting* out . . . and *coming* out.

There is another advantage to an outdoor shape-up . . . it's a great way to meet new men. The two best ways? Running with a group and joining a health club. Both are filled with men who are as conscious of the way that they look as they are of how the women look. One thing to keep in mind, however, is that if you are truly going to work out at a gym, or really get into running, you have to take it seriously.

Writing a large check to a health spa doesn't count as exercise. If you join a health club, you should take advantage of the exercise, and not the crack manicurist. And just because you own several hundred sweat suits, don't think that you're automatically in shape. Wearing sweats won't do you one bit of good . . . especially if you wear them to drive to the fast food place to load up on fried chicken and those little cardboard apple pies.

So, start with your most resistant muscle . . . your brain. When it says sit, you say sit-ups . . . when it says walk, you say run.

Now, let's take a look at the way the rest of humanity shapes up.

Running Away from Home

GET READY

Everyone, it seems, is running . . . away from their own flab. But before you start to run, you should walk. Take your cues from kids, in fact. Watch children: first they walk and then they run. Begin by walking to build up stamina. Then incorporate walking and jogging. Start out with two minutes of walking, followed by two minutes of jogging. If you can do this for twenty minutes without collapsing, you are ready to become a runner.

But before you do, get yourself a good pair of running shoes. Your shoe should be specifically designed for running. If not, you could end up with wrecked feet and undue muscle strains. At the beginning, run on flat surfaces only, and use a heel/toe motion, even though it may seem unnatural at first.

GET STRETCHED

You can't run well if you haven't stretched well. So begin and end each running session with exercise . . . about ten minutes worth before and five minutes worth after you run.

And stretching your muscles is one of the most important things you can do. Begin with wall pushups . . . they are great body stretchers. Then do as many of each exercise as you can.

- Stand about one-and-a-half feet from the wall, with palms flat to the wall. Lean forward with heels planted firmly, and hold for ten seconds. Relax. Start with ten to stretch the hamstring muscles.
- To stretch your Achilles tendon, lean forward against a wall with your fingers pointed toward the ceiling. Then slowly walk backward from the wall, keeping your heels flat to the ground.
- Touch your toes. If you can get your palms flat to the floor, that's even better. Don't bend your knees and don't cheat. Start with ten toe touchers.

AND GO!

Runners know that different running regimens require different running disciplines. For example, for short sprinting you need power. For distance you need endurance. If you're not used to strenuous exercise, it's important that you build your body up for the chase. Don't expect to get out the first day and run too far for too long. Begin with nonpercussion training. Regular workouts in a pool, on the exercycle, or even cycling on the street can help to tone your body, without too much stress. And beware of overstress once you've established a running routine. You may notice the onset of soreness in certain areas, or a change in your running style. For example, a smooth run may become a gallop rhythm. If this happens, stop your running routine until you see a physician.

Added stress on these body parts can halt your running program permanently, unless treated.

The Weighting Game

Okay, so you say running isn't for you. Then how about weight training? For sure, you will meet lots of men *that* way. (We're talking about men who work out in coed health clubs, not muscle-bound crazies who can't bend their arms anymore!) But even with the men in the health clubs, you have to take it seriously.

While it's true that men who are working out love to watch women working out, you'll have to earn your keep . . . they expect you to be one of the boys . . . they don't expect to give up their time to help you constantly. So, if you want to work out alongside of them, you should know what it's all about.

WHO, WHAT, WHY WEIGHTS

Weights are great for flattening the stomach and trimming the waistline and the upper arms. Weight *training* as opposed to weight *lifting*, which is a professional sport, is also a great way to strengthen your body for whatever sport you play.

But if you are resistant about weight training, because you think it will make you muscle bound—forget that: It won't because it can't. The male hormone testosterone is responsible for a man's short, bulky muscles,

Women simply can't become as muscular. Then why do some women athletes appear muscular? Because these women work out six or seven hours a *day*. We're talking about working out two or three times a *week*.

Basically, there are three types of weights for weight training. Free weights are the traditional dumbbells and barbells, which you may or may not find at your health club.

Then there are weight machines. One type, the nautilus, is actually a group of machines, each designed to exercise a muscle group. Another, the universal gym, is a multi-exercise device that tones all of the muscle groups.

Health clubs, "Y"s, and gyms can help you to get started on the weight-training program that is right for you. You might pick up any of the books out now on the subject. Diana Nyad's *Basic Training For Women* from Harmony Books is a good one to get acquainted with.

But, however you begin, be careful because you might get hooked. It's really fun and who can resist being the only female in a room full of half-naked men? Not I!

I'm Dancing as Fast as I Can—Dancers' Tips for Staying in Shape Through Dance

Dancers have great bodies. You know that. But did you know that even dancers have to work at keeping themselves in shape, while keeping their energy level up?

Well, if you've decided that a dance class is probably easier than weight training and more fun than running down the street with large dogs chasing you and small children laughing at you, read on. These tips are from Marion Horosko, beauty and fashion editor of *Dance Magazine*.

• Before you decide to starve yourself and plunge into dance simultaneously, remember calories measure the energy you expend. Take a tip from the previous section and calculate your daily calorie needs. Then add on a bit more if you are seriously dancing every day.

• Dancers drink lots and lots of liquids, eat foods rich in protein, snack on fresh fruits and veggies, and limit their intake of salt and sugar. So should you.

• After class, nibble on potassium-rich foods like oranges, bananas, or fruit juice.

• You *can* work out too hard . . . and then become dehydrated. Professional dancers actually weigh themselves before and after a performance. They make up the water loss (which is *not* a weight loss, incidentally) by drinking water at regular intervals until they've gained back the difference.

Bonus dancer's tip—If you've a got a long drive or hike ahead of you, do as dancers always do, and stop drinking fluids two hours prior to departure. But keep half a lemon handy. It will quench your thirst and give you a vitamin "C" boost to boot!

You may find that dance is just the perfect exercise for you. But more importantly, you will find that with a sensible combination of diet and exercise, you'll start slimming down with out slowing down.

WHAT ARE YOU WEARING TO THE DANCE?

If dancing is the way you choose to go, take these tips from the pros at Danskin, so that you're not in a whirl about what to wear.

- *Thinking about ballet?* Ballet dancers prefer professional weight nylon tights worn with layers of leg warmers. (leg warmers keep muscles warm, which prevents leg cramping).
- *Modern dance?* Footless tights let you exercise your innovative moves in bare feet (no slipups).
- *Jazz dancing?* Pack up nylon Lycra jazz pants, leotards, fishnet hosiery, and jazz oxfords.
- *Aerobic dance?* Opt for cotton leotards or T-shirts and shorts with sneakers.

FIGURING OUT WHAT'S BEST FOR YOUR FIGURE

Well, it's all great and terrific for women with perfect proportions in perfect portions, you say? Well, no one's perfect you know. Here's how to disguise what you've got too much of, and bring out what you've got too little of.

- *Legs too short?* Look for leotards with high-cut legs . . . and your legs will look much longer.
- *Narrow shoulders?* Look for cap sleeves.
- *Small bust?* Look for gathers in the front.
- *Large bust?* The simpler the better is the key to your look. Stay away from shirring, gathers, horizontal banding at the bust.

And remember, dance clothes do double duty. You can always dress them up and take them out to dinner. So choose the prettiest clothes you can find. They will make you feel like a star . . . even if you're a falling star at the beginning!

KEEPING TRACK: COUNTING UP THE CALORIES AS THEY BURN AWAY

The following is a list I've compiled of many of the outdoor or away-from-home exercises that you might consider doing. Let's take a look at how efficient each one is at burning up calories. This list is based on a person weighing 120 pounds.

Sport or exercise	Calories burned per hour
Badminton—singles	310
Basketball	495
Bicycling (10 mph)	370
Calisthenics	
Light	245
Heavy	585
Dancing	225
Golf (9 holes, 2 hours)	225
Handball	695
Jogging (5½ mph)	585
Jumping rope	455
Skiing	530
Cross country skiing	625
Stationary Bicycle (10 mph)	375
Swimming (30 yards per minute)	375
Tennis	380
Walking (3½ mph)	280

CELLULITE: GETTING RID OF THOSE HATEFUL DENTED THIGHS

Are you a prisoner of cellulite? Who isn't? Cellulite, which shows up as the lumpy bumps on thighs, bottoms, inner knees, and God knows where else, has been called a fad word for fat. Cute, but that doesn't help you if you never could resist fads. Many doctors who've done research on cellulite have stated that cellulite is actually no different from ordinary fat . . . it is simply fat that localizes in specific areas. Others state that cellulite is a combination of fat, water, and wastes, which is trapped under the skin in "pockets."

But whatever it is, or isn't, if you've got it you don't have to be stuck with it. Well, you probably know whether you've got it, but you might not know whether you're about to get it . . . or actually whether it's about to start showing. Here's how to tell: Pinch a bit of flesh on your thigh, buttocks, or wherever you suspect that cellulite might be showing up. Squeeze gently. If it looks more like cottage cheese than a leg, you've got it. Now, let's get rid of it. There are three basic ways to do just that. Let's take a look:

The Nutritious Way

You are what you eat . . . that's for sure, and cellulite not only is what you eat, it sometimes even looks like what you eat. Good nutrition and a well-balanced diet can really help a great deal in getting rid of cellulite. Here are the foods that you should eat more or less of:

- Cut down on fats and starches. Get your carbohydrates from natural fruits and vegetables.
- Stay away from extra seasoning and cheeses . . . especially cellulite's lookalike, cottage cheese.
- Drink lots and lots of water. At least eight to ten glasses a day. This will help to flush your system of the trapped fat and water. The more water you drink, the more you flush your system.
- Other foods to avoid: Sugar, butter, soft drinks.
- Suspected villans include: Cigarettes, diuretics, and lack of exercise. So get active! Jane Fonda doesn't have dents, does she?

The Friction Method

The other way that works, especially in conjunction with a good program of nutrition and exercise, is the friction method. Products such as the Methode Elancyl, which consists of a hard plastic mitt with a bumpy underside of rubber, is used in the shower or bath. By following the directions, you simply massage the offending areas with the soap-filled mitt. After you step out of the shower, simply apply the special cream. The method works by encouraging the trapped fat to circulate. It really does work, too. In fact, I, who was *born* with cellulite, began using this method a few years ago. A plastic surgeon whom I was dating (whose entire business it is to spot flaws) mentioned to me when we were at the beach one day, that I was the only woman he'd ever seen without any cellulite. I, of course, turned around to see who he was talking to. But he wasn't speaking to anyone else . . . he was talking about me! It really *was* gone! But, remember, the minute you stop using these methods, the cellulite will come back. So this is more or less a lifetime commitment. It's worth a few minutes a day to be without oatmeal legs.

The Surgical Method

The final method of getting rid of cellulite is a fairly new surgical procedure called lipolysis, according to Dr. John Grossman, a plastic surgeon in Denver, Colorado. This is a technique in which the localized fat is surgically suctioned out through a small incision on the area.

The incision, which is usually no bigger than two to three centimeters (about an inch), allows the surgeon the space needed to insert the suctioning tube. The procedure is done under general anesthesia and requires about a three-day hospital stay.

The disadvantages to this type of surgery? Dr. Grossman feels that there just haven't been enough of such operations performed for surgeons to know whether or not surgery is the right answer in every case.

The results, however, can be quite dramatic. The size of the thighs, buttocks, even ankles can be reduced. But he also points out that deformities cannot be removed, and once the skin shape has been established, it cannot be reversed.

How long does it last? In general, the surgical changes are permanent, but remember, your body will nonetheless react in much the same way that it would had the surgery not been performed. For example, if you've had a face lift, you will still age. Similarly, with lipolysis, if you gain weight, you can gain it back there. But since fat cells are actually removed, there would be a somewhat lesser weight gain in the areas of the surgery.

18 · Clothes Makers

COMING OUT OF THE CLOSET

You are now ready to get up and almost ready to get going, so let's take a look at what you've got to wear. Take everything out of the closet. Yes, everything, including shoes, hose, belts, bags, scarves, undies . . . EVERYTHING! Now, try everything on. Then try them on in combinations that seem insane. You will be very surprised to learn that the sweater you haven't worn in three years looks wonderful with the cotton dirndl skirt that you bought by mistake.

    Try to be as wild as you dare. Remember, no one is looking and no one is there to laugh. Then put aside everything that absolutely does not fit. You know which things they are. I know that it's hard to admit that the cutoffs you wore in high school have finally stretched beyond the point of human endurance, but THEY WILL FIT AGAIN SOON.

First, put everything that no longer fits (but that you love) in a box and label it HOPE CHEST. Then box up everything that you haven't worn for three years or more (give away only what you really hate) and save anything that has possibilities for making a comeback. I have thrown away or given away more clothes that I wish I had now than I care to admit. Remember, the leather mini skirt you bought in the sixties, which made you look like a Hell's Angel in the seventies? Well, if you gave yours away like I gave mine away, it will cost you $300 to find it again and be chic in the eighties!

Now, put everything back together in the closet. You can either hang all of the clothes together by category, such as all shirts, all slacks, or you can hang them in combination the way you will be wearing them.

For example, let's get back to that sweater and dirndl skirt. If you've suddenly made a great discovery of how to put these items together, you might hang them together with the scarf and accessories that you'll be wearing them with. This truly speeds up dressing time, and makes you feel extremely organized. It's just what the high-priced fashion consultants tell their clients to do. And it may indeed work for you.

If you've discovered nothing else with this closet expedition, you've discovered that you needed to clean out your closet anyway, and you've probably found the umbrella that you swore the painter stole.

Seriously, what you have discovered are some very important things about yourself. Are you hanging on to a style of dress that was important to you at a time in your life when you were happiest? Well, that doesn't mean that it can make you happy any longer. Are your clothes from the past bright, for example, and your clothes today, all in neutral shades?

Take a look and evaluate whether the clothes you've purchased have been at times in your life when you were happy or sad. The sad clothes probably look that way.

Then decide which clothes just make you FEEL terrific, and which ones make you feel dumb, uncomfortable, or unsure of yourself.

Put away the clothes that make you feel dumb or insecure. If you feel that way, even if you don't look that way, you'll project an uncomfortable image. And right now, you need to feel self-confident, not self-conscious.

You will be able to take those clothes out again in a few months, when your confidence is back, but just don't wear them now. Really.

So what you've got left is a basic wardrobe of clothes that look well on you and make you feel great. You also have a few boxes full of future potentials, and a very clean closet. That in and of itself should give you a boost! See, I told you I wouldn't force you to go out!

CLOTHES ENCOUNTERS: HOW TO HIDE EVERY POSSIBLE FIGURE FLAW

You don't have to be fat or skinny to have a figure problem or two that needs a bit of camouflage. And wearing the right clothes can not only create an illusion of perfection, but also can make you feel as good as you look. Remember, we are at the confidence-building stage of your makeover now. When you start going out into the arena again you should look and feel sensational. And you will.

Here's another story. My affair was kaput, my time was up, and I had to go out. So I accepted a date with a very boring rich person (it was safe). He invited me to a major party (800 people) at the estate of another boring rich person. When I went to the closet, like Mother Hubbard, I found it bare! Just nothing was right. So, I went out and bought a dress that certainly wouldn't have suited me in my previous incarnation. (I'd always tended to wear clothes that made a statement). But the dress that I bought this time was just a long strapless slip of black silk. I topped it off with a gold shawl that my mother crocheted for me. That was it (besides a pair of diamond studs in my ears).

I was five pounds thinner than when I was in love, my hair was in great shape from the months I had spent lying around conditioning it, but most of all . . . I felt pretty. And my dress was *perfect* for me. It showed off my new slimness, and hid the fact that I still didn't have great legs. I felt so dazzling that I not only kept Mr. Boring happy, but I also managed to mesmerize a whole table's worth of men! I went home with several dates, several enemies (women who actually got angry with me because their dates were flirting), and a whole new outlook on myself.

But, most importantly, I learned a very valuable lesson about myself. I realized that when I get myself in shape, I don't need gimmicks. Now *I* wear clothes . . . they don't wear me. I've traded in trendy for elegant, stylish for individuality. Now my clothing makes the most of what I've got and hides what I've got too much of. So, that party showed me something I won't soon forget. Simple is not only better . . . it's a knockout! Remember, elegance always beats trendy for drop dead glamour!

WHAT TO WEAR WHEN THERE'S TOO MUCH (OR NOT ENOUGH) OF YOU

Have you ever looked into a funhouse mirror and decided that *those* proportions were more to your liking than your real ones? Well, if you aren't thrilled with what you've got, and don't have the time to wait until you get what you want, here's how to instantly dress into what you'd like to have. After all, you need to feel great right this minute . . . you *are* going out, you know.

Hiding It All

• Optical illusion can create, if not a slimmer you, then a slimmer-looking you. Remember, vertical or diagonal stripes carry the eye upward, giving you a thinner, taller look.
• Look for slenderizing fluid lines (No! Not tent dresses, please! They just make you look older and pregnant). Shawl collars, dropped waistlines are good slimmers too . . . as are softly tailored suits with contrasting blouses. And you can go for the bright lights in the blouse.
• Deemphasize hips with A-line and dirndl skirts.
• Large breasted? Keep yourself in balance by sticking to simple, uncluttered necklines. Do just the opposite if your breasts are small.
• Keep a long line going by matching panty hose and shoes in the same dark tones.
• Keep an eye on fit . . . it's the most important thing you can wear. Check your clothes for gaps and puffs in the back.

- If you still need to lose a lot of weight, try a half size, and buy *one* outfit only. Remember, you want to look wonderful today. You can always throw it out, when you are at your goal weight. A half size can give you the look of a custom fit . . . which adds chic to your style.
- Choose slim, unbelted shapes that emphasize necklines, sleeves, or cuffs.
- Go for collarless blazers that cover your bottom.
- Pair jackets with sleeveless blouses. You don't need that extra bulk under your jacket.
- You know the old adage: "If the shoe fits wear it." But did you know that if the pants won't, don't? Size nine pants on a size twelve body won't help you to look slimmer, but will, in fact, call attention to the problem areas. Clothing should skim, not cling, to the body.
- Fabrics, too, are important. Choose flat, woven fabrics in silk, cotton, and knit. Avoid bulky tweeds. And please, please, please stay away from glitter and stretch. If you want to wear them now, don't. But keep in mind that you will, and very soon. You are already well on the way to letting the skinny person who's been hiding inside of you come out. Right?

Best Breast Bets

Too ample in the bosom? Too sparse in the blouse? Then take heed, and take these clues. Please.

- If you are tall and bosomy, don't worry about anything. You'll have relatively few problems, because your long torso will let you carry long lines.
- If you are short and bosomy, however, your large

bosom can dominate the whole upper half of your body. So, keep away from any style that shortens the torso, such as wide belts and high waistlines. Tight-fitting tops were for Lana Turner . . . they're not for you. Instead wear loose-fitting tops with gathered shoulders that are simple in design.

• If you are big busted you simply must spend the extra money for a good bra. An ill-fitting bra cannot only destroy a great fashion look, it can also destroy your shoulders.

• Too small on top? Actually your fashion silhou-ette presents relatively few problems. And besides, you've got a much better chance of keeping gravity at bay for a much longer time. But if you do want to create the image that less is more, go for horizon-tal stripes, gathers, high waist styles.

A Quick Rundown of Other Problem Spots

• Broad in the beam? Best disguisers are high-waisted, flowing dresses, full or A-line skirts, and pants that are cut straight from the hip.

Bonus tip—Fullness in cut should always start at the widest part of the hips.

• Shoulders too small? Stay away from collarless styles, big lapels, halters, raglan sleeves. Choose, instead, crisp fabrics, soft shoulder pads, set-in sleeves, dolman sleeves, and gathers at the shoul-ders. Steer clear, too, of puff sleeves and horizontal designs. Instead choose raglan sleeves.

The Long and Short of It

How much do you know about the long and short of it? Do you know, for example, that the longer *you* are the longer your jackets can fall, because you can afford to cover some of your leg and still appear stately? If you're short, however, a shorter jacket will give a longer look to your body. Your waistline, too, is an important consideration when you choose your clothes. If you're short waisted, you should stay away from wide belts. If you wear them at your natural waistline, they end up right below your bustline, leaving too little torso and too much belt. The one exception to the rule is a stiff, wide belt that you wear right below your natural waistline. Pull it tight so that it won't shift, and you've created the illusion of length.

Think that your waistline is too long and legs too short? Then stay away from low-rise pants and do look for high-rise trousers and high-waisted skirts. High heels also add length to your legs. Finally, have the hem of your pants fall to the instep of your shoe tip. Keep the line from your waist to your shoe as long as possible.

Short Stories: Dressing Tall

If you'd like to look a few inches taller, you can achieve the look you want with a few basic tricks. First, to add an illusion of more height, get a long line going. It's the one rule of dressing "tall" that can help you to break the other rules. So try to keep the shoulder to hip line one color or the waist to toe line one color. It's important, too, to pull the eye to the extremities. If you're really tiny, go for a bright color at the neck or the feet. If you love skirts, but don't want to break up the line, keep your shoes and hosiery in the same shade as your skirt. And when you shop, remember that stores run out of the small sizes quickly, so shop early. And remember, too, that you have the run of the boys and preteen departments. But keep it simple, not childish.

Tall Stories: Dressing Small

The trick, if you're tall, is not to look like you go on forever. How? Go for layers and bulky necklines. You can wear them. Fill in V necklines with scarves or turtlenecks. Try wide shoulders and bold slashes of color at the waist with bright belts that cut you in half. And don't be afraid of color! It's yours to play with. When you shop, keep in mind that stores run out of large sizes quickly, too. So shop early. Shop the men's departments for shirts and sweaters. You should be concerned with buying investment clothing because good clothes allow more alterations than cheaper garments. Also since you may be spending more on alterations, you want the clothing to last from season to season. So, if you're tall, just remember the basics: good proportions, long jackets, lots of textures, and huge accessories. Now, that's a real tall story.

Suiting Up to Suit Your Shape

Okay, here you go, it's time to get out. Maybe you've joined a health club and all you see lolling around the pool are wonderful men. Or maybe you are a beach lover and God knows *what* you've found. But you're worried . . . you suspect that you may be showing too much you and not enough suit in too many of the wrong places.

Well, you say, there's nothing you can do about that. A swimsuit just won't disguise figure flaws, right? Wrong.

In fact, a swimsuit *can* disguise flaws *and* build up assets. So keep these tips in mind before you go shopping for a suit to suit your needs:

• If you tend to saddle bag in the hips, but want to wear a high-cut maillot anyway, choose one that has an inverted V leg in front rather than on the sides. This will draw the eye away from the problem area and onto the assets.

• Other hip tips? Choose a swimsuit without special hip detailing. Avoid gathers, shirring, horizontal stripes, and loud prints. Look instead for a suit that flattens (and tightens) and one that gives you ample coverage in the seat.

• Full busted? Look for support definition under the breasts. And stay away from details that overemphasize your overload. Things to avoid like the plague include shirring, tucks, gathers, or horizontal bands of color. And make sure that there is ample coverage on the sides of the cups . . . especially if you intend to swim in your swimsuit.

• Small breasted? Avoid suits that flatten you out. In this case, go for what the fuller breasted woman can't wear . . . gathers, tucks, pleats, horizontal color bands, and tank suits.

• Small bottom and hips? Make the most of it. You can actually wear anything your little heart and your little hips desire. But bikinis are made for you.

• If you are wide, go for vertical patterns and stripes.

• Want an overall slimming swimming suit? Then remember that strong colors and busy prints are not as slenderizing as softer color combinations.

Danskin's line of TrimSkins® actually hold you in like a lightweight girdle. And while they're trimming, they look sexy and gorgeous. I own several. They are even great at supporting large breasts without all of that awful armor.

• And no matter what your proportions, remember that suits with high-cut legs, give a longer line, while V necks lengthen the neck and flatten the bustline.

• Pear shaped? Look for horizontal details up top . . . it will give the illusion that less is more, and that more is less, bringing your whole body back into proportion.

• Midriff crisis? Then choose blouson styles that don't hug the tummy.

• Choose a strapless suit if you are only interested in tanning. For swimming, you need a suit that stays put. Pretzel and T backs and all variations on the competition suit are your best choices. Otherwise, you may end up not only a fallen women, you may end up a woman with a fallen suit.

THE LAST WORD ON WARDROBE

After you've gone through all of the other considerations for your wardrobe, let's get to the big one—money. While it might be all well and good that you've found your look, it doesn't help if you can't afford it. (And who in these inflationary times can?) Here are some keys to help you unlock a too-tight fashion budget:

Begin by building a classic wardrobe. This, however, takes foresight and tunnel vision. It's much too easy to be swayed by fads and trends. Don't. If you want to look trendy, you can always jazz up a classic look with kooky accessories. My recommendation is to begin with a good blazer. Even if your budget only allows you one purchase this year . . . make it a blazer. A blazer can be teamed with classic wool, flannel and cotton skirts and pants, or it can be worn over a dress or even over a dazzling nighttime ensemble. The main thing about a blazer is that it is interchangeable. It can go to work during the day and go out dancing in the evening.

Keep your shoes and handbags in neutral colors, too, so that they can transcend the seasons, if not the years. For the bright spots, which make your clothing special, buy bright scarves and belts in wild designs and colors. In fact, one of my favorite fashion tricks is to tie a giant chamois square scarf over a very classic outfit. Instant identification.

Here, then, a bunch of things that you can do with one really good black blazer:

- Pair it with a pleated skirt or gray flannel trousers for work and you're all business.
- For a sleek sporty look, that same blazer can be teamed with a turtleneck sweater, an oxford shirt, or even a silk blouse and a pair of your favorite jeans.
- Be creative! You don't *have* to put that blazer away when summer arrives, you know. You can use it in place of a boring sweater on cool summer nights. It's a knockout with a white T shirt and white duck pants, or even with pleated top shorts.

So, if you've got lots of ideas, but not lots of money, buy less, but buy better. It pays!

Investment Dressing

How can you tell if a garment is worth the investment? Well, one thing we all know, in this the world of sixty-dollar blue jeans, is that a price tag doesn't always assure quality.

Look not at the price tag, or whose name is displayed on the outside of the garment. That's right, turn it inside out. See if it looks as neat on the inside as it does on the outside. Check the pressing. Make sure that there are no wrinkles where the sleeve and the shoulder line meet. Check the button holes. Are they perfectly executed? Then check the buttons. Better clothes have better buttons. You'll see buttons made of mother of pearl, leather, and horn, rather than plastic. Good dresses just don't have plastic buttons . . . or belts. But if a dress does come with a belt of matching fabric, or even plastic, switch it to a leather, rhinestone, or medallion and cord belt. Then it's uniquely yours.

Blend with the Trends

But what about those expensive things you've already got hanging in your closet? You know, the ones that just are "that much" out of style? Well, the good news is that you've got this year's wardrobe already hanging in your closet . . . you just don't know it. The trick is to revamp and recycle!

For example, last year's pleated top trousers can become this year's pegged-leg baggies by simply tapering the leg. Or they can be transformed into a pair of right-this-second bermuda shorts or middy pants with a few well-placed snips and stitches.

The bottom line, then, on deciding what to recycle

and and what to toss is quality. Fine-quality fabrics, such as cashmere, silk, good wool, and good cotton, are just naturals for recycling.

Accessory Aficionado

Accessories are wonderful. I love them. And the best part is that they can be CHEAP, CHEAP, CHEAP, and no one will ever know.

To make even the most classic look come alive:

• Shop the thrift shops, and look for the outrageous. Antique fur pieces, such as those forties scarves with heads and tails, are spectacular for dressing up a tailored suit.

• If you can find it, snap up a fur boa, too. Last year I bought a silver fox boa, which is six feet long, for seventy-five dollars in a thrift shop. I see them selling in the exclusive fur salons for thousands now. But what can you do with such an item? Have a great time, that's what! I use it as a boa over strapless evening wear at night, and a scarf over a suit or coat during the day. It's pure knockout when you enter a room for a dressy dinner in a black fitted suit and a silver fox boa. Again, the unexpected.

• Look, too, for antique evening wear. The fabrics are usually sensational, and the styles will knock you off your feet. So will the prices. You can usually find a great dress in the fifty-dollar range.

• Check out the thrifty bargains in antique costume jewelry, and evening bags, too.

• Stalk the closets of your mother, aunts, and grandmother. There's no telling what you'll find.

• Don't discount the five-and-dimes, either. You

can find great cheap accessories like big plastic button earrings, headbands, jelly beach sandals, combs, ribbons, pretend diamond stud earrings (if you wear them once or twice per pair, and toss them out, no one will ever know you're wearing paste, not posh).

• Hats. Buy them by the carload and wear them constantly. They can be a great trademark for you. Again, look into the antique and thrift shops for straw and felt hats. Look, too, for glittery hats and veiled hats. They are too sensational to pass up . . . if you've got the nerve to wear them.

19 · Getting Over the Agony of Defeat

VENTURING BACK OUT: HOW TO MEET MEN

Now that you know *how* to look, and how to look *out* for the wrong kinds of men, it's time that you thought about what kinds of men you want to *look* for. Even though you still might not be 100 percent, it's time that you started testing the waters, and seeing just how your new good looks work.

But, before you get out, there are several things that you should know. The first and most important thing about getting over a good relationship that went bad is that you cannot continue to direct your energies toward the negative. If you keep wallowing in the past, you will simply destroy your future. You've had your chance to wallow, and now it's time to live again. Too much wallowing will make you bitter and more unhappy than ever. Your relationship is over, and it's time that you got on with living and finding a newer, more satisfying one. Believe me, at some point in the near future you will meet someone, and be amazed that you ever cared about Mr. Once-Was in the first place. It does happen, you know.

But how and where do you meet this new one? Well, you probably won't meet him in your house, that's for sure. The only place where you'll stand a worse chance of meeting someone than in your house, is in a bar. Think about it this way: Would you want to become friends with a woman you met in a bar? Then why should you subject yourself to meeting men that way?

So let's rule out singles bars right off the bat. They are just what the name implies: bars for single—eternally single—people. And besides, why should you force yourself to become part of the meat rack? It's demoralizing and the odds are stacked in the men's favor. Think not? Then think about this: Do men look desperate to "find" someone in a singles bar, or do they look like thay are cruising for the best possible piece of meat they can find? Why should you be rated by nerds you wouldn't even want to have lunch with, let alone get involved with!

And the reality is that you always do better when it's just you and a man . . . not when you're in an environment that breeds competition. You are simply stacking the cards against yourself to compete with a roomful of other women.

How then do you meet men? The best way is still through friends. Friends can fix you up with friends, friends have parties where there will be men (and other women, it's true, but it's still friendlier than a bar), And friends, especially married friends, like to see everyone paired off. So bug them, cajole them, haunt them if you need to, but get them to introduce you to men whom they think you'd like.

Another good way to meet men is to take classes that you think you'd enjoy and classes that you think men would enjoy. For example, photography courses are the kinds of classes that newly divorced men sign up for. It has something to do with spreading their wings and being creative.

Investment courses are good, too. Men who are making it (but obviously are not in banking) need to learn how to handle their money, right? Besides, you need to learn how to handle your money, too. It's a primo meeting ground.

There are also courses given all over the country on the financial strategy of divorce. Even if you have never been married . . . go. A man who's worried about getting taken to the cleaners at least has enough money to worry about. And while it's true that it's as easy to fall in love with a rich man as it is a poor man, rich men are a whole lot harder to find. So if that's what you want, hang out where they hang out. You can always date the instructor if worse comes to worst.

But what if you are already divorced or have never even been married? How do you justify your presence to someone you'll meet? Tell him that you are taking a law course and thought that this would be an interesting addendum to it. Or tell him that you are doing a free-lance article on divorce. If, however, you are in the midst of a divorce, take one of these courses for sure. Even if you don't meet anyone, at least you'll learn what your rights are.

Another good way to meet men is to attend sporting events. These arenas are the only places in town where on any given Monday night, the men outnumber the women fifty to one. Now that's the kinds of odds I like. But pick your sport carefully. If you want to meet average middle-income guys, you obviously wouldn't go to the polo matches, and vice versa. The two sports that cross all economic barriers are, of course, football and baseball, although soccer is a close third. Hockey is a real hit and miss. I've known really wealthy guys (desperados) whom you can find at a hockey game one night and the opening night of the opera the next. But hockey attracts a lot of men's men, and a lot of families. (Men's men, by the way, are the men who hang out and drink with their friends . . . and would rather do that than anything else.)

Another classic way to meet men is to fly whenever you can to wherever you can. And fly first class whenever possible. The compartments are smaller and the men are usually better. Another sure fire *guaranteed* way to meet men is to fly rather than drive to the best weekend place in your part of the country. The men who fly to their summer houses are guaranteed to have two things: (1) They have a second car, which they keep just for the weekends, which means that they probably own their houses; and (2) They are too busy to buck traffic with the rest of the sweltering masses.

I've a friend who flys to her rented (and shared) house every weekend. She never spends a weekend alone. She meets them by the planeload every Friday on her way out and she meets them again on the Monday morning flight back. Of course, she, unlike most of the rest of us, can afford to do that. If you can't, at least plan to do it once or twice during peak season (even if you have to skip going out to dinner for a while to do it).

Especially hot runs on the Eastern seaboard are the Friday night and Sunday night flights between the Hamptons and LaGuardia airport (the Marine Air Terminal). The flights that are even hotter than those are the

TransEast and P.B.A flights between New York and Martha's Vineyard and Nantucket. Any time after 4 P.M. on Fridays and any time after 6 P.M. on Sundays and early Monday mornings are the hot tickets to get.

But alas, a hot ticket does not a vacation make if the hot ticket is to the wrong place. So find out the best possible places to get to in your area, then rent a house (even if you have to coerce every person you know into sharing it with you), and then spend as much time as you can there.

Now, Nantucket, as we've mentioned, on the East Coast is very special because not only is it gorgeous, but it has more than just blues and stripers running, it has men running! In fact, on any given week between July and August you can find more men then you'd find at homecoming at West Point.

But if Nantucket is simply not an easy commute for you, then do try places that are. For example, you might try Newport in Rhode Island (rich, well educated, WASPY), Vail in Colorado, Park City in Utah, Port Arthur, Texas, Ketchum, Idaho (for winter skiing), Hilton Head in South Carolina, and, of course, places like Lake Tahoe, Steamboat Springs, Marina Del Rey, and Laguna Beach on the West Coast are always hopping.

Now, if you are looking for something completely off the beaten track, you might even think about a place called Harbor Point in Michigan. This is a little island with large houses. The people who come here for the summer actually have enough money to not be kidding when they ask each other where they plan to winter! Well, at any rate, there are some very interesting men who "summer" here in their "cottages," which are usually large versions of the White House, and these "cottages" have been in their families longer than their families have even existed. If you can possibly get to this

---

strange place, then stay in the town outside the "private" area. Chances are good that you will find the man of your dreams just sitting around waiting for the buggy (there are no cars on the roads, just a horse-drawn carriage with driver) to pick him up to take him out of Harbor Point so that he can talk to someone about something other than where she plans to "winter".

Meeting men in the winter, of course, requires different tactics. So take a writing course in off-season and then get assignments interviewing men whom you'd like to meet. (Or at least men with professions that seem interesting to you.) I'm serious. I've met more men that way than any other way.

Actually it's perfect. You are the only woman in the room and you get to do all of the asking. I've never left an interview without a date, unless I wanted to. Even if you take a journalism course at night, you'll get assignments to interview people. People rarely say no because they are flattered by the gesture.

Other good ways of meeting men, as we've mentioned earlier, are health clubs and sports clubs. If you join a health club, however, you will be in competition with other women, so do what they *aren't* doing. Get into weight training and become one of the boys . . . they'll see how much of a woman you are in no time . . . flat. Besides, if you don't become involved with any of these men at least you'll become friends, and they will have friends, you know.

Are you a runner? Organizations and clubs for runners are great places to meet men. You'll not only stay in shape, you'll get to meet men who share your love of running. The bonus? You'll become quite friendly with the men you run with, without the single's club stigma.

Which brings up another good point: Cultivate your male friends. Men make terrific friends, and can be great for you now. They do things like put up shelves, go to the movies, and hang around with other men. Lots of women I know have met new men through old male friends. It works. Besides, male friends are great to talk to, don't put any demands on you, and work really well as escorts when you need to go to the company Christmas party with a date.

Particularly wonderful are gay male friends. They make the best companions because you never have to worry about having them make an unwanted pass. And when you go to a party with a gay friend, you get to flirt with every man you want to, while having a date, and offending no one.

Other more conservative, but reliable ways of meeting men are, of course, the zoos and the museums on Sunday. Divorced men always resort to these places when they don't know what to do with the kids. It helps if you bring a child along. My daughter always runs off and plays with the other kids at the museum and at the zoo. And I always end up talking with their parents.

Another great meeting ground is a large men's store. One woman I know has had phenomenal luck at Barney's in New York on Saturdays. Barney's is one of the biggest men's stores in the world so she gets to shop for whatever kind of man she's attracted to by going directly to the department that carries his kinds of clothes. She's met a banker in the preppy department, a professional hockey player in the Izod shop, and a doctor in the formal wear shop. But how does she do it? It goes something like this:

She spends time agonizing over a shirt or tie or something (in the formal shop it was a cumberbund and matching bow tie, which she now wears). She then turns to the man she's been eyeing and says something like, "If you were my brother, would you like this?" It works every time. She works Barney's while the rest of the women in New York are agonizing over where all the men are! She usually scores pretty well, too. The hockey player even bought her an Izod shirt and had the clerk send it based on the name and address he'd accepted on her check. They began dating and it lasted for several months. I knew that the relationship was in trouble when we had lunch on a Saturday and she told me that she had to make it quick because she needed to get over to Barney's to buy her father a shirt.

And, of course, you should never overlook the limitless supply of live ones at the local political clubs. Now, at least fifty percent of these men are married. Of that fifty percent, probably half are there because they believe in the system and the party, and the other half are there *to* party . . . away from their wives (lest we forget "The Eternally Married Man, on page ——)

But, aside from the married ones, there are a lot of other men. Some are boring go-fers, who like to rub elbows with the elite. Some are really smart guys with good minds and better bodies. And, aside from being assured of meeting men, you'll be getting into a new circle where you'll have the opportunity to go to parties with lots of new people and generally find something to get excited about again. You may even decide that instead of joining 'em, you'd rather beat 'em and run for office yourself. It's sure worth a go!

Finally, don't be afraid to take risks. One of the most fun men I've dated I met at a party because I was willing to take a risk. He was seated at my table and we were both with dates. It so happened that both of our dates had left the table at the same time. He asked me what my last name was and I looked him right in the eye and said, S-T-A-S-I, "and it's in the book." He laughed and said, "I'll call you." I said, "When?" And he said, "What time are you getting home?" It was really romantic and clandestine. He loved it. I loved it. And we had fun together, although we never got around to loving each *other*.

So take those risks. Remember, you look wonderful now. And even if you can't get to Barney's to meet men, they *are* everywhere, you know. If you are nervous, begin by striking up conversations on elevators . . . if you are afraid of rejection, you don't have to wait long for him to disappear.

Be bold. Have fun. Use lines. I love telling men that they are unique and special. In fact, I simply use the best lines that men have used on me, on them. It works.

Malcolm Forbes, among others, has said that the only things to regret are the things you never try. He, who's made a very successful life for himself, said that if he tried and failed, at least he wouldn't think that he could have been successful at something and wasn't. Make that your philosophy, too. Feel good about yourself, and learn to collect men the way that men collect women. Don't think of every date as a potential marriage partner. And don't turn down dates because you know that it will never lead anywhere. I used to think, "How can I have dinner with you when I don't want to marry you?" I don't think that way anymore. Now I go out with lots of men. I've gotten over the fear of being uncomfortable about the sex thing. If they make a pass, and I am not interested, I simply say that I am celibate. It works every time, as I have mentioned in the beginning of the book. They think at first that they will be the ones to change my ways, and will give me time. And do you know what? By that time, we've already become friends, which is more important than the sex. And no one's feelings are hurt. Men just don't want to continue dating you if you tell them that you aren't interested in them sexually. It's demoralizing for them and embarrassing for you. This little fib keeps everyone happy. It is, after all, your body and your life . . . learn to take control of both. You needn't do anything with either of them that you don't want to do!

REVENGE IS SWEET: THE STORY OF ULTIMATE REVENGE

And now, the ultimate revenge story. What you are about to read is true; only the names have been changed to protect the not-so-innocent.

Carol was the untiring wife of a man who was in law school. Carol, as the old story goes, was working *his* way through law school. She suffered through his bouts of depression and worry over the bar exam, his constant nitpicking at her, his poking fun at her "tight-fisted" ways. Behind her back, Arthur used to say, "Well, even if she is a dog, she certainly is a loyal little pup." Arthur was not a nice person.

In fact, when Arthur finally got his first job at a prestigious law firm that specialized in criminal law, he proved how unnice he truly could be. After all of that struggle to get him through, now it was Carol's turn. Or so she thought. On the night she announced to Arthur that they were going to have a baby, he answered her by saying that he had forgotten to tell her that he didn't want to be married anymore!

He said, in fact, that he'd fallen madly in love with a female psychiatrist who'd testified (more like lied) on behalf of one of Arthur's clients. She was brilliant, he said. She'd convinced the court that Arthur's perfectly sane client, who had murdered someone, truly was insane. "Instead of life in prison, my client got a term in the loony bin," he boasted. Arthur was quite crude.

Out the door went Arthur without another word. Carol, on the other hand, had many words. She did, in fact, drive everyone within a hundred-mile radius crazy with words. After a time, however, Carol decided to stop sitting around mourning her loss. She'd go out and make something of herself. After all, if she could make something of Arthur, she could make something even better of herself. God knows, she had a lot more to work with. And so she did.

While Arthur and his live-in shrink were living high on the hog, Carol was living at her mother's, raising a baby, going to medical school, and working part-time doing insurance physicals. But finally she made it. She became a doctor and a successful one at that.

When she was ready for it, she had a friend, who was a plastic surgeon, fix her nose and give her a chin implant. She bought new clothes, changed her hair style and color. She was now not just a successful doctor, she was a gorgeous one. Finally, she was having the life she'd really wanted. She had millions of men, lots of fun, a great house, a terrific kid. And that's the end of the story, right? Not quite. Carol, you see, got to experience the ultimate revenge.

One day about ten years after good old Arthur walked out without a word, Carol's phone rang. She picked it up and guess who it was?

Arthur, it seems, had gotten himself into a bit of a scrape and sure could use Carol's help. (He secretly knew in his heart that she'd come through, loyal lap dog that she was.)

You see, as luck would have it, Arthur's second wife, the shrink, had gone and gotten herself a lover. She didn't find Arthur nearly as exciting after they married as she had while they were living together, he explained. Well, he didn't like that one bit, so he began secretly following wife number two and her lover. Whenever (and wherever) he found them he would make a scene . . . sometimes in public. It was perfect. So number two and her lover, who was, incidentally, also a shrink, concocted a scheme. And before he knew what was happening, Arthur himself was committed to a loony bin. Number two was quite crude, too. But heaven knows she'd had enough experience committing the sane to the insane places.

Carol was Arthur's only way out. At least *she* knew that he was sane, right? He asked Carol (after a ten-year/no child-support-silence) to come by the hospital and get him released. And, oh yes, would she mind picking up a fresh suit of clothes for him on the way? He knew in his heart that Carol had never *really* forgotten him. And it was true. She hadn't. She *had* been waiting for him to finally come to his senses . . . or to lose them completely.

She waited. And when Arthur finally asked for help, she said: "Sorry Arthur, I've got a Tupperwear party to go to!"

Carol then packed up a suitcase. Her own. She was, you see, on her way to St. Tropez with the world's handsomest man.